Non-Suicidal Self-Injury Throughout the Lifespan

A comprehensive guide for clinicians working with patients engaging in self-injury, this book provides information on clinical conceptualization, risk and protective factors, ways to assess for NSSI, treatment approaches and strategies, and early intervention and prevention strategies.

Focusing on ethical and cultural considerations unique to schools, clinical agencies, and private-practice settings, the authors provide a practical and in-depth discussion of clinical theory. Procedures for determining risk and the potential problems with risk assessment, especially concerning suicide risk, are addressed. In addition to numerous exercises, examples, and suggestions for practical interventions, the book includes a variety of detailed worksheets and resources to expand readers' level of understanding, monitor emerging trends, and provide a context for extended training. Several case studies are discussed and analyzed in order to highlight specific aspects of clinical conceptualization and treatment strategies.

Drawn from a wide range of treatment populations and issues, this book is a valuable resource for clinicians and supervisors. The authors integrate outcomes-based research strategies and evidence-based tools to help clinicians work with clients from diverse backgrounds.

Kelly Emelianchik-Key, PhD, LMHC, NCC, ACS, is a licensed clinical mental health counselor and assistant professor in the counseling department at Florida Atlantic University. She has completed extensive research and training in teen dating violence, non-suicidal self-injury, and sexuality issues.

Amanda La Guardia, PhD, LPCC-S, NCC, is a licensed professional clinical counselor supervisor and assistant professor for the counseling program at the University of Cincinnati. She has completed extensive research and training in the areas of non-suicidal self-injury and suicide, gender-related issues, and professional development.

"This book is a vital addition to the literature on non-suicidal self-injury (NSSI). Our profession has been riddled with misunderstanding about this behavior in clients we serve. This text offers clarity on the subject and also offers us multiple treatment plans and interventions. It outlines NSSI across life development stages, which offers a unique perspective in the discussion of self-injurious behaviors. The case studies provide information and assistance that will be vital in working with clients who have a relationship with NSSI. I applaud these authors and have deep appreciation for what they have added to the literature in our field." — **Patricia E. Robertson**, EdD, professor emerita, East Tennessee State University, USA

"Emelianchik-Key and La Guardia have produced thorough and timely guide for practitioners and students who need effective guidance in treating the complicated issue of non-suicidal self-injury. With practical tools, detailed case studies, and thorough treatment strategies, this guide will become an important reference tool for any clinician." — **Paul R. Peluso**, PhD, LMHC, LMFT, professor and chair of the Department of Counselor Education, Florida Atlantic University, USA

"NSSI is one of the most pervasive and destructive activities among adolescents and young adults, so you would think that there would be a ton of useful information on the people and processes, both individual and systemic, that are affected by this problem. Sadly, this was not the case—until now. This book brings all of us up to date on the problem and its treatment in a very readable text that is loaded with case studies. As a person who has experienced this with a family member, I can say without hesitation that I wish this book had been available ten years ago." — **James Robert Bitter**, EdD, NCC, past president of the North American Society of Adlerian Psychology, professor of counseling and human services, East Tennessee State University, USA

"Emelianchik-Key and La Guardia expertly guide readers through the complexities of NSSI, weaving in available best practices, resources, and scholarship from across the helping professions. The authors provide an innovative, thoughtful, and case-based approach for assessing and treating diverse clients across the lifespan with NSSI. This text is a must-have clinical resource!" — **Danica G. Hays**, PhD, professor of counselor education and executive associate dean, University of Nevada, Las Vegas, USA

Non-Suicidal Self-Injury Throughout the Lifespan

A Clinician's Guide to Treatment Considerations

Kelly Emelianchik-Key and
Amanda La Guardia

Routledge
Taylor & Francis Group
NEW YORK AND LONDON

First published 2020
by Routledge
52 Vanderbilt Avenue, New York, NY 10017

and by Routledge
2 Park Square, Milton Park, Abingdon, Oxon OX14 4RN

Routledge is an imprint of the Taylor & Francis Group, an informa business

British Library Cataloguing-in-Publication Data
A catalogue record for this book is available from the British Library

Library of Congress Cataloging-in-Publication Data
A catalog record has been requested for this book

ISBN: 978-0-8153-7134-2 (hbk)
ISBN: 978-0-8153-7135-9 (pbk)
ISBN: 978-1-351-20359-3 (ebk)

Typeset in Goudy
by Nova Techset Private Limited, Bengaluru & Chennai, India

Kelly—This book is dedicated to all of the clients I have worked with over the years. Your bravery to share your stories and the courage you show is inspirational in more ways than you will know. I am appreciative of the amazing colleagues and mentors that I continue to learn from and work with, especially my co-author and friend Mandy. One of my favorite Robert Frost poems has a line that says, "Two roads diverged in a wood, and I, I took the one less traveled by, and that has made all the difference." To my husband and family, thanks for always giving me support, love, and encouragement to take the road less traveled. Thank you to my kids; your presence and love motivate me to make a difference.

Mandy—This book would not be possible without the tireless efforts of my co-author and the experiences I've had with colleagues and clients over the years. I hope this book honors the stories of the clients I have had the distinct privilege of working with and learning from. Special thanks to Patricia Robertson, who helped me to understand the importance of self-reflective empathy and cultural humility when working with self-injurious clients; thank you for encouraging me to grow as a practitioner and, foremost, as a person. Thank you to my daughter Aria, with whom I get to practice being my better self.

Contents

PART III
Ethics and treatment of non-suicidal self-injury

PART IV
Worksheets and resources

Preface

We decided to write this book in response to a growing need for clinically focused, easily understood guide for treating individuals engaging in non-suicidal self-injury (NSSI) that includes an interdisciplinary perspective. Through our work, we have noticed the increasing need for more practical ways to approach NSSI and to help clinicians working with challenging cases that can be difficult to conceptualize. NSSI is a complex issue, and no two cases are identical. Due to this diversity, it can be challenging to produce consistent findings in research studies, which means evidence-based practices are difficult to pinpoint.

Through this book, we hope to offer some information that will be helpful for clinicians as they attempt to address the concerning treatment issues related to self-directed violence to include NSSI and suicidal behaviors. In this preface, we intend to define important constructs related to self-directed violence that will give you some background information on the terminology that is important in NSSI research. This book will be broken up into three main sections. Each section intends to highlight issues that may intersect with specific developmental concerns across the lifespan. Many complex client issues are presented in cases within the first three chapters of this book, which we will follow throughout the other chapters.

List of figures, tables, cases, and textboxes

Key terminology

Literature reviews and searches on NSSI can be difficult due to the numerous terms that can be used to describe NSSI, but there are also many definition discrepancies that may exist in the literature (Mangnall & Yurkovich, 2008). The following terms will be discussed and defined per recent peer reviewed literature, CDC, and DSM 5 criteria. These are the definitions that will be used throughout this book. As you will notice, many of the definitions and terms overlap, which makes NSSI even more complex and difficult to conceptualize when examining confounding variables within research.

Self-directed violence (SDV)

Self-directed violence is an umbrella term that incorporates a broad range of violent behaviors, including fatal and non-fatal suicidal behavior or acts, non-suicidal intentional self-harm (i.e., behaviors where the intention is not to kill oneself; NSSI). It also includes suicidal ideation (i.e., thoughts about, considering, or preparation for suicide), even though it is not a behavior due to the connection to self-directed violent behavior.

- *Non-suicidal self-directed violence*: Behavior that is self-directed and deliberately results in injury or the potential for injury to oneself. There is no evidence if it was implicit or explicit, of suicidal intent.
- *Suicidal self-directed violence*: Behavior that is self-directed and deliberately results in injury or the potential for injury to oneself. There is evidence, whether implicit or explicit, of suicidal intent.
- *Undetermined self-directed violence*: Behavior that is self-directed and deliberately results in injury or the potential for injury to oneself. Suicidal intent is unclear based on the available evidence.
- *Suicide attempt*: A non-fatal self-directed potentially injurious behavior with any intent to die as a result of the behavior. A suicide attempt may or may not result in injury.
- *Interrupted self-directed violence—by self or by other:* Other—A person takes steps to injure self but is stopped by another person prior to fatal injury. The interruption can occur at any point during the act, such as after the initial thought or after onset of behavior.

By self (in other documents may be termed "aborted" suicidal behavior)—A person takes steps to injure self but is stopped by self prior to fatal injury.

Crosby, A., Ortega, L., & Melanson, C. (2011). Self-directed violence surveillance; uniform definitions and recommended data elements. Retrieved from https://www.cdc.gov/violenceprevention/pdf/Self-Directed-Violence-a.pdf

Self-harm (SH)

Operational definitions of self-harm can vary, but most often include the intentional or purposeful acts of non-fatal self-poisoning or self-injury, most are often without intent to die and have a non-fatal outcome.

Latimer, S., Meade, T., & Tennant, A. (2013). Measuring engagement in deliberate self-harm behaviours: Psychometric evaluation of six scales. *BMC Psychiatry*, 13(1), 4.

Suicide

Death caused by self-directed injurious behavior with an intent to die as a result of the behavior.

- *Suicide attempt*: A non-fatal, self-directed, potentially injurious behavior with an intent to die as a result of the behavior; might not result in injury.
- *Suicidal ideation*: Thinking about, considering, or planning suicide.

Centers for Disease Control and Prevention (CDC) (2018). Definitions of self-directed violence. Retrieved from https://www.cdc.gov/violenceprevention/suicide/definitions.html

Non-suicidal self-injury (NSSI)

The self-inflicted tissue damage that is intentional, direct, socially unacceptable, and without suicidal intent (e.g., cutting or burning the skin, self-hitting, self-punching or hitting)

Nock, M.K. (2010). Self-injury. *Annual Review of Clinical Psychology*, 6, 339–363.

The International Society for Self-Injury Research defines NSSI as the following:

1. First, the harm that results from self-injury is an *intentional* or *expected* consequence of the behavior. Risky behaviors that could result in harm, such as not wearing a seatbelt while driving, or accidental harm, that may occur when playing extreme sports, are typically excluded in our definition.
2. Second, self-injury usually results in some sort of immediate *physical injury*, including cuts, bruises, scratches, or marks on the skin. Behaviors that do not directly result in injuries are usually excluded, even though they may be harmful or dangerous. For instance, food restriction is typically not considered a form of self-injury since the associated physical damage tends to build up over time instead of happening all at once when the behavior occurs.

3. Third, self-injury is separate from suicidal thoughts or behaviors, in which individuals want to end their lives. People usually report that they have no expectation or intention to cause death when they engage in self-injury. In fact, in some cases, self-injury may be used to manage intense distress that may be associated with suicidal thinking.
4. Finally, behaviors that might cause physical damage but are acceptable in our society, or part of a recognized cultural, spiritual, or religious ritual, are not considered self-injury. For this reason, body modification, body piercing, or tattooing are not usually considered forms of self-injury.

Retrieved from
International Society for the Study of Self-Injury. (2018, May). What is self-injury? Retrieved from: https://itriples.org/about-self-injury/what-is-self-injury.

Deliberate self harm (DSH)

Deliberate self-harm, sometimes also referred to as non-suicidal self-injury, is defined as the intentional or deliberate, direct destruction or modification of body tissue without conscious suicidal intent or thoughts, which results in injury that causes tissue damage (e.g., scarring).

Gratz, K.L. (2001) Measurement of deliberate self-harm: Preliminary data on the deliberate self-harm inventory. *Journal of Psychopathology and Behavioral Assessment*, 23, 253–263.

Self-injurious behavior (SIB)

Non-accidental and self-inflicted acts that cause damage to or destruction of body tissue and are carried out without suicidal ideation or intent. Again, used synonymously with NSSI.

Nock, M.K. (2010). Self-injury. *Annual Review of Clinical Psychology*, 6, 339–363.

Self-mutilation (SM)

Deliberate, non-suicidal destruction of one's body tissue, which sometimes occurs in such culturally sanctioned practices as tattooing; body piercing; and healing, spiritual, and order-preserving rituals. SM can also include head banging, self-biting, trichotillomania, and skin picking.

Favazza, A.R. (1998). The coming of age of self-mutilation. *The Journal of Nervous and Mental Disease*, 186(5), 259–268.

Para-suicide

This term is intended to be a broad term to describe all non-fatal self-injurious behavior with clear intent to cause personal harm or death, thus leaving "attempted suicide" as the term where the intent of death is clear and known. An example would be a sublethal drug overdose or slashed wrist.

Bille-Brahe, U., Schmidtke, A., Kerkhof, A.J., De Leo, D., Lönnqvist, J., Platt, S., & Sampaio Farla, J. (1995). Background and introduction to the WHO/EURO Multicentre Study on Parasuicide. *Crisis: The Journal of Crisis Intervention and Suicide Prevention*, 16(2), 72.

Emotional dysregulation (ED)

Not having control not only over how and when, but also the intensity, of emotions that are felt, experienced, and expressed.

Gross, J.J. (2002). Emotion regulation: Affective, cognitive, and social consequences. *Psychophysiology*, 39(3), 281–291.

Interpersonal-psychological theory of suicide (IPTS)

Developed by Thomas Joiner, this model attempts to explain when some people engage in suicidal behavior while others who are at risk do not. The presence of thwarted belongingness and perceived burdensomeness must come together with acquired capability for suicidal desire. Thwarted belongingness is a painful emotional state when someone's needing to connect with others is not met. Perceived burdensomeness is how much someone feels like they take a toll on others around them and is often the mindset of "person X would be better off if

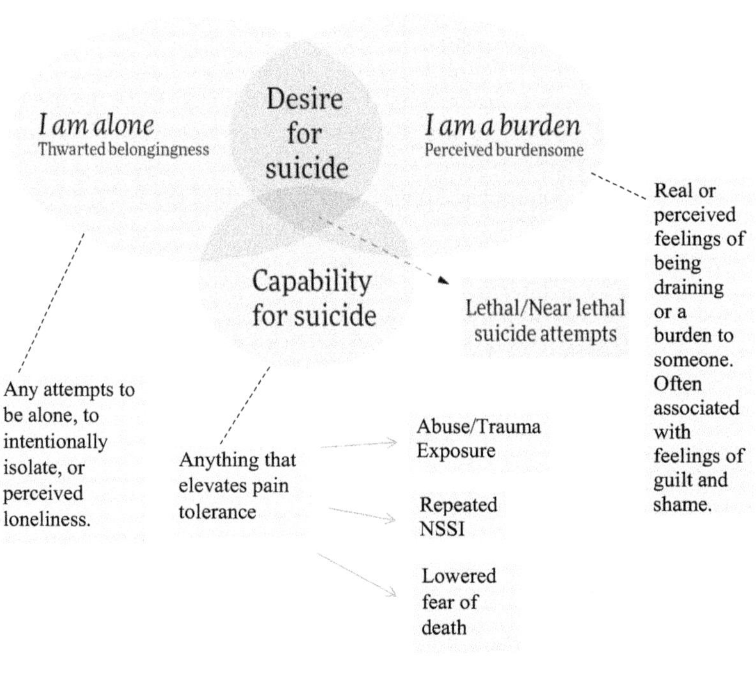

Figure A Joiner's interpersonal theory of suicide.

I were gone." Acquired capability is the ability to withstand pain. This is where NSSI comes into play. If someone feels like a burden and also does not feel like they belong, continued engagement in NSSI could eventually lead to suicide. The longer someone self-injures, the more pain they can tolerate. Eventually, the same cuts or burns are not enough to take away these negative psychological feelings and turn to suicide. See Figure A below.

Joiner, T. (2005). *Why People Die by Suicide*. Cambridge, MA: Harvard University Press.

Ethics statement

We appreciate all clinicians' ongoing endeavors to help their clients overcome non-suicidal self-injury. Non-suicidal self-injury is a complex topic, and there is no one way to go about working with a client. We have attempted to provide as much comprehensive information in this book as possible to assist you on your journey toward helping clients reach their goals to stop self-injuring and above all to remain safe. However, we do want to remind you that there is no quick fix and information is continually changing, evolving, and progressing in NSSI research. Remember always to practice within your scope of professional practice and your area of competence and expertise. Make sure that you follow all of the ethical and legal guidelines in your given profession and, if in doubt, always consult with other experts, colleagues, and professionals who can help you make the most appropriate clinical and ethical decisions when working with your clients.

Authors

Kelly Emelianchik-Key, PhD, LMHC, NCC, ACS, is a faculty member in the Department of Counselor Education at Florida Atlantic University. She received her Bachelor of Science degree from Florida Atlantic University, Master's and Educational Specialist degrees in Mental Health Counseling from the University of Florida, and her Doctorate in Counselor Education from Old Dominion University.

Dr. Emelianchik-Key, has experience working with diverse populations. She has spent a great deal of time in various roles working with complex traumas, dating violence, behavioral issues, and self-injurious behaviors in clinical and non-clinical populations over the last 15 years. When she is able, she works with a small caseload of adolescent and adult clients in private practice. Dr. Emelianchik-Key is an engaged member of the counseling community via her work with clients, teaching, research, providing clinical supervision, serving on editorial boards, writing and publishing, and her work within national counseling organizations. Her areas of research interest and clinical expertise include dating and intimate partner violence, self-injurious behavior, clinical supervision, gender issues, work with marginalized populations, sexuality and intimacy issues, and ethics.

Amanda La Guardia, PhD, LPCC-S, NCC, is a nationally certified counselor and a licensed professional clinical counselor supervisor in the states of Texas and Ohio, with past licensure as a professional counselor in the state of Tennessee. Dr. La Guardia has worked in the mental health field since 1999 beginning with a summer student worker position at Western Psychiatric Institute in Pittsburgh, PA. Since then, she has held a variety of roles at differing levels of care within state-funded and private contracting agencies. Dr. La Guardia has over 10 years of experience in community mental health that involved collaborative planning and care with both juvenile justice and school systems, which brings a useful perspective on the inter-relationship between mental health concerns and their effects on the family, schools, and greater community as well as the importance of interprofessional treatment modalities. She specializes in working with children and families experiencing cyclical crisis, symptoms related to trauma experience, and suicide-related behaviors (i.e., non-suicidal self-injury/self-directed violence). Since 2009, Dr. La Guardia has published articles in professional peer-reviewed journals in medicine, counseling, and psychology on topics related to gender issues in counseling, suicidal behaviors, non-suicidal self-injury, interdisciplinary approaches to the treatment of health concerns (e.g., insomnia), and other practice issues. Dr. La Guardia currently maintains a small private practice and works as a counselor educator at the University of Cincinnati.

Contributing Authors

Ellen K. Chance, PhD, is a certified school counselor for Florida Atlantic University (FAU) Lab Schools in Boca Raton, FL. Dr. Chance works with a diverse 9th–12th grade student population enrolled in an early college program. She also serves as the coordinator of the K–12 comprehensive school counseling program, FAU High School near-peer mentoring program, and school-wide social-emotional learning programming. Her areas of specialization include counseling children and adolescents, crisis response and intervention, social-emotional learning and development, and improving student connectedness through the delivery of a comprehensive, data-driven school counseling program. In addition to her work as a school counselor, she enjoys serving as an adjunct counselor educator and supervisor. She presents nationally on topics related to child and adolescent anxiety, social-emotional learning, and comprehensive school counseling.

Mariah Dern, LPC, is a student at the University of Cincinnati, pursuing her doctorate in Counseling Education and Supervision. Mariah received her master's degree in counseling from Cincinnati Christian University and a bachelor's degree in Family Science from the University of Kentucky. She has experience working with clients anywhere from high school aged to adulthood, from substance use disorders (SUDs) to severe and persistent mental illness (SPMI), and from private practice settings to community mental health. Her favorite part of the profession, though, is to teach, supervise, and work alongside new counselors entering the field.

Bridget Glass graduated from Palm Beach Atlantic University, in West Palm Beach, Florida, with a Master of Science in Counseling and is currently pursuing a doctoral degree in counselor education and supervision from Florida Atlantic University. Her work as a counselor and educator has spanned over 15 years, affecting children from infancy through adolescence. Additionally, Bridget is an advocate for victims of domestic violence and provides community training on the mental health impact of trauma on survivors and their children. Bridget is trained in both Eye Movement Desensitization and Reprocessing (EMDR) and client-centered play therapy. She resides in Jupiter with her husband of 18 years and their two fluffy Goldendoodles.

Adriana Labarta, LMHC, MEd, EdS, is a doctoral student at Florida Atlantic University's Counselor Education and Supervision program. Clinically, Adriana is passionate about working with individuals with eating disorders and has experience treating diverse clients in residential, partial hospitalization, intensive outpatient, and college counseling settings. Her therapeutic approach focuses on providing a safe space to promote both acceptance and change for individuals in recovery. She is an active member of the American Counseling Association and the Association for Counselor Education and Supervision. As a future counselor educator, Adriana intends to further contribute to the counseling field through research, teaching, supervision, and advocacy work.

Part I

Introduction to client case scenarios

In this section, case studies emphasizing aspects of non-suicidal self-injurious behaviors throughout the lifespan will be introduced. These case studies will be detailed and used throughout the book to highlight specific aspects of clinical conceptualization and treatment strategies. We intend the inclusion of integrated case studies to provide the reader with concrete examples that demonstrate the complexity of clinical decision-making in relation to NSSI and to provide a clear process by which the theories and research presented in the text can be applied. There will be a "what-if" dialogue that will be used throughout that will be important for the reader when considering different treatment outcomes. The dialogue will also help the reader to understand how the scenario might change if the client presents with different cultural or situational considerations. This contextually based approach will assist the reader when utilizing the information in their practice.

1 Non-suicidal self-injury in childhood

Kelly Emelianchik-Key

Self-directed violence in the form of non-suicidal self-injury (NSSI) occurs in approximately 18% of the pediatric population worldwide (Muehlenkamp et al., 2012) and is a strong predictor of an eventual suicide attempt (Andover et al., 2012). Suicide is the second leading cause of death for children, adolescents, young adults, and adults between the ages of 10–34 years old (CDC, 2017). NSSI is considered a pervasive issue among the adolescent population, but there is limited information about self-directed violence in children under the age of 14 (which includes both suicide and NSSI). However, there is strong evidence that children as young as seven years of age are engaging in forms of self-directed violence (Barrocas et al., 2012).

Early childhood development

When working with younger clients who engage in NSSI, it is important to first begin by examining developmental theories and the unique role they play in self-injury onset and engagement. Developmental theories most often divide childhood through stages that are marked by quantitative differences in the child's behavior and development. Erik Erikson's psychosocial developmental theory (1963) is one of the most well-known developmental theories. Eight stages divide the lifespan, which focus on changes in social interaction and growth through development. Each stage is marked with challenges that people commonly face in that stage of development. If not addressed appropriately, these challenges can impair growth, possibly for a lifetime. Jean Piaget's (1976) theory of cognitive development divides development up into four stages, which define cognitive processing by age. Table 1.1 below breaks down each of the stages. In each of the cases presented, the clients are posed with challenges that can prevent or impair their cognitive and developmental stages. When working with clients engaging in NSSI, it is critical to assess these stages. This can assist the clinician in tailoring their treatment plans and picking the most appropriate intervention strategies.

Table 1.1 Piaget and Erikson stages of development

Piaget stage of cognitive development	*Outcome*	*Erikson' stages of psychosocial development*	*Conflict*	*Important events/people*	*Virtue*	*Outcome*	*Positive resolution*
Sensorimotor Ages 0–2	**Senses and motor responses coordinate. There is a sense of curiosity about the world. Learning is achieved by looking, touching, and sucking. Interaction with the environment takes place.**	**Infancy** 0–18 months	Trust vs. Mistrust	Feeding Parents	Hope	A sense of trust is developed when constant, reliable care is provided and affection is given. Without this mistrust forms.	Security
		Early childhood 18 months–3 years	Autonomy vs. Doubt	Toilet training Parents/ caregiver	Will	A sense of control is formed over physical skills and independence. Success leads to feelings of accomplishment and autonomy, and failure results in shame and doubt.	Feelings of independence
Preoperational 2–7 years	**Symbolic thinking takes place and language is used for expression. Egocentric thinking and imagination grow.**	**Preschool** 3–6 years	Initiative vs. Guilt	Exploration Parents/ teachers	Purpose	Control is asserted over surroundings. Success leads to feelings of purpose, and those who fail by exerting too much control experience disapproval and guilt.	Balance between impulsiveness and control
Concrete operational 7–11 years	**Logic is used, and interpretations are made in relation to concrete objects.**	**School Age** 6–12 years	Industry vs. Inferiority	School Teachers/ significant others	Competency	New social and academic demands are presented and children who succeed in this feel competent. Those who do not feel failure.	Self-confidence

(*Continued*)

Table 1.1 (Continued) Piaget and Erikson stages of development

Piaget stage of cognitive development	*Outcome*	*Erikson' stages of psychosocial development*	*Conflict*	*Important events/people*	*Virtue*	*Outcome*	*Positive resolution*
Formal Operational 12–adulthood	**Abstract thinking begins, and hypothetical ideas. Reasoning begins to take place.**	**Adolescence** 12–18 years	Identity vs. Role Confusion	Social Relationships Friends	Fidelity	A personal sense of self and identity is formed. Success leads to ability to feel confident about one's self, and failure leads to role confusion and feelings of inferiority.	Unified sense of self
		Young adulthood 19–40 years	Intimacy vs. Isolation	Romantic Relationships Community	Love	Intimate and loving relationships are formed with other people. Success leads to strong relationships, and failure leads to loneliness.	Form close personal relationships
		Middle Adulthood 40–65 years	Generativity vs. Self-absorption	Workhood, parenthood, coupling Community	Care	Adults look to nurture and create things that are lasting and will create positive change. Success leads to feeling useful and accomplished, while failure leads to feelings of defeat and lack of competence	Promote others' well-being
		Maturity 65+ years	Integrity vs. Despair	Reflection of life	Wisdom		Sense of satisfaction with a life well lived

Youth who engage in NSSI are best suited to individual and family counseling, as these are the most appropriate treatment options, given that the culture of the home is largely structured by caregivers. Being exposed to increased levels of childhood family adversity and trauma exacerbates NSSI behaviors due to the added stress and is viewed as a trigger and risk factor for adolescent NSSI (Fliege et al., 2009). The automatic functions of NSSI, such as the ability to regulate affect, self-punishment, and peer connection components, directly relate to adverse childhood experiences (Kaess et al., 2013). This further supports the involvement of family members in the treatment of NSSI in children and adolescents. In this chapter, we present two case studies involving youth who self-injure. Each case will serve to present the clinical decision-making process from assessment to conceptualization of NSSI behaviors and treatment modalities. We review cases from male and female biological sex categories because NSSI behaviors have been shown to present differently for individuals identifying as male or female, particularly in youth. Intersections of diverse experience and group identification are also explored in each case. Experiences with societal and cultural stressors linked to identity can influence the emotional experience of the individual engaging in NSSI as well as their treatment needs associated with the behavior.

Case 1.1: Case of Jenny

Jenny is a 9-year-old, multiple-heritage female. She reportedly has a good relationship with both of her parents; however, they reside in different homes in the same city. Her father identifies as bi-racial (African American and Asian), while her mother identifies as White. She has two younger siblings, ages four and two. Jenny's parents separated two years ago and have been divorced for about six months. Jenny has a history of hitting herself and hair pulling. Around the age of six, Jenny's parents noticed that she would bang her head on the floor and inconsolably cry when she became frustrated. They thought Jenny was having trouble with changes in the home and figured that the behaviors would pass. Then, around the age of seven (following the separation of her parents), both of Jenny's parents noticed that her eyebrows were thinning, and she appeared to be pulling hair out of her head while she did homework, as well as on days when she moved from one parent's house to the other. Jenny's parents have tried different methods to stop the behaviors, but they have become increasingly frustrated. Jenny has a large group of friends at school and seems to fit in with everyone. She is popular in her peer group. Jenny's parents say her teachers report they have not noticed self-injurious behaviors at school. Her teachers note that Jenny is a hard worker and tends to help other children in her class. She is also active in after-school soccer and seems to enjoy it. When at home, Jenny helps to watch her siblings as much as she can and tries to be caring. Jenny's mother says that she sometimes notices behavioral problems when she asks Jenny to complete a task. Jenny can become visibly frustrated if she does not do it "just right." Jenny visits her father every other weekend and for one month in the summer.

Jenny's dad ignores the hair pulling and expects Jenny's mother to attend to the behavior and "make Jenny stop." When Jenny tries to bang her head or hit herself, her father says he restrains her and punishes her. He states he does not notice the behavior as much as Jenny's mom does and wonders "how much it really happens." Jenny's mom believes the self-directed violence is just part of a phase, but she frequently tries to talk to Jenny after an incident to make sure she is calm and convince her to stop the behaviors. Jenny's parents argue quite a bit about what to do when Jenny has difficulty. Both indicate a desire to help Jenny. When asked about her self-injuring, Jenny becomes frustrated: "I'm tired of talking about this. My mom and dad need just to leave me alone. My mom is overreacting, and it's not a big deal."

Developmental perspective

Jenny's behaviors began to appear at a critical age. In Erikson's developmental theory (1963), Jenny would be in the industry v. inferiority stage. Typically, in this stage, a child's world expands at school, and social interactions play a critical role. This stage is where children begin to feel accomplished and confident. They start to take pride in the tasks that they complete. The most impact usually comes from encouragement by adults around them, typically from parents and caregivers. Additionally, at age five, most kids begin school and enter a structured kindergarten/educational setting. This is where teachers begin to take on another critical role for children. For most children, this new atmosphere will change their normal routines. The transition to school also brings about different educational and social expectations for children. Jenny entered school around the same age that her hair pulling began. This is important to note since there were many critical factors going on at one time during this age for Jenny. Jenny built new peer relationships and has begun to gain academic expectations. This can bring about stress and anxiety for some children. Jenny needs to have a balance of encouragement and support from her teachers. She also needs to feel unconditional love and support from parents. Jenny is doing well in school, which tells us that she is getting what she needs while at school and feeling accomplished and competent as a student. This is critical for her developmentally. Additionally, working with Jenny's school and making them aware of the NSSI behaviors can be helpful for Jenny's treatment progress. The school can support Jenny's parents by having specific and detailed self-injury protocols and maintaining open communication about Jenny's behaviors. Encouraging an open dialogue with teachers and staff not only best supports the student, but also assists the school in understanding the safety concerns that exist for the student.

During the same time that Jenny began school, a new sibling was born. Upon the birth of a new child, parents typically become preoccupied with additional parenting responsibilities. Parental time with Jenny became split between her and another child. When considering developmental tasks at the onset of the self-injurious behaviors, one might consult the Eriksonian task of competency.

In combination, introduction to a new school environment, adjusting to a new sibling and changes within the family dynamic, and new expectations related to academic performance and peer relationships can create significant stress for a child. During the period between ages six and eight, children usually begin to learn more appropriate ways of effectively expressing and talking about thoughts and feelings. Leading up to a phase in which emotional development becomes a greater focus for social adjustment, Jenny was consumed with changes that may have been overwhelming for her. Her inconsolable crying and headbanging evidence this assertion, as both coping strategies began at age six. These self-destructive actions are a common method for young children to display non-suicidal self-injurious behavior (Klonsky, 2007). Whereas most children this age would verbally express frustrations and emotions regarding the environmental stressors, Jenny's method for coping is to engage in NSSI behaviors to have some control over the situation and cause more turmoil.

Another significant transition occurred when Jenny was seven, namely the separation of her parents. Divorce and separation can present a difficult transition for children, changing emotional and physical support and needs related to safety and belonging. Divorce can be a major risk factor for children, particularly related to internalizing and externalizing problems. As a clinician working with Jenny, it would be important to assess how cooperative co-parenting is going and the ways conflict is managed in relation to Jenny. Child-parent relationships are negatively affected by childhood family adversity (Hughes et al., 2004), and can be a precursor and risk factor for childhood and adolescent NSSI (Fliege et al., 2009) and other internalizing/externalizing issues (Lamela et al., 2016). At the onset of NSSI, Jenny's parents did not seek professional assistance, nor did they directly address Jenny's changing emotional needs related to home and school changes. During the time following the onset of NSSI, her self-destructive behaviors expanded to include hair pulling. Moving between homes and additional challenges associated with her parents' separation appear to have overwhelmed Jenny emotionally. Her expressivity of feelings was not typically verbal or verbally processed at home and was often demonstrated through her actions (self-directed and disruptive).

When considering Jenny's behavior in relation to her home environment, sibling relationships might also need to be assessed to determine the level of family involvement in treatment. Just before the separation of Jenny's parents, another sibling was born, potentially creating a lot of disruption in the home. During this time, Jenny would've been preparing for or transitioning to second grade and entering into a period of significant cognitive development (concrete thinking), thus limiting her thinking to what she perceives as real based on experience without consideration of possibilities (abstract thinking). A child of this age could believe that the addition of a new sibling would bring about the same types of changes in the home as occurred with the previous sibling. Jenny may perceive any shift away from her experience-based expectations as being attributable to her parents increasing focus on her coping behaviors (it is possible she blames herself and is potentially punishing herself).

Given the developmental links to the realization of self-esteem, self-confidence, and a need for emotional support, parental involvement is essential to the treatment of issues associated with Jenny's use of NSSI and the reduction of self-destructive behaviors. Her father appears to have an authoritarian parenting style, marked by strict expectations, punishment, and little room for collaboration and emotional support. Children from authoritarian homes are at higher risk of developing self-esteem issues and tend to have difficulty managing anger felt toward the authoritarian parent. Jenny's mother appears to display a permissive style of parenting. She encourages Jenny to talk about the NSSI as well as what is bothering her, potentially demonstrating that she takes the problem seriously. However, she fails to encourage alternative ways of coping and fails to address potential issues in the home contributing to the behavior. She also seems to communicate a simple message concerning the behaviors: "stop." Children of permissive parents can also have low self-esteem, report excessive sadness, and at times do not respect authority or rules. The contrast in parenting styles could be leaving Jenny feeling frustrated and emotionally overwhelmed. One's own experience as a child often influences parenting styles and how those experiences are perceived in relation to one's identity and cultural values. Thus, addressing approaches to parenting can often be difficult within the context of counseling. A clinician must balance understanding and empathy with challenging the family in order to focus on first- and second-order change. Family counseling and parenting training would be very beneficial for working on the issues concerning Jenny's NSSI behaviors. The counseling could address the meaning of culture and how to best work with Jenny and her parents in relation to her cultural identity. There are also many negative feelings, worry, blame, and confusion, about how to respond to a child's behavior of NSSI, which can lead parents and caregivers toward hypervigilance and the use of authority and power to try and take control (Kelada et al., 2016). These actions can worsen family functioning and increase NSSI behaviors (Baetens et al., 2015). Family counseling would also be an outlet to discuss best parenting techniques and ways to help parents and caregivers navigate Jenny's behaviors. For more information on parenting resources, see Appendix A.

Lastly, a focus on developmental strengths is important for the development of a treatment plan with Jenny. Jenny appears to have strong social relationships at school and is also able to respond well to stressors within the school environment, as self-destructive behaviors have not been observed at school. While the need for perfection with Jenny's performance seems to create emotional turmoil at home, it has not presented as an issue at school. Perfectionism can be a predictor of increased anxiety levels, and thus, while Jenny may be experiencing anxiety at school, she does not engage in headbanging or hair pulling. While increased performance anxiety could be influencing Jenny's NSSI behaviors, she can healthily manage them. The counselor would need to explore more about her personality and determine the role that perfectionism plays in her life. It would also be important to explore her people-pleasing behaviors, need to be helpful in various environments, and what appears to be a need to be liked by others. All of these needs are developmentally typical and could serve as important internal supports and motivators, but they may also be presenting barriers for Jenny, depending on how she perceives herself (self-esteem and competency/ability). Being well liked may help her self-esteem, but it may also increase pressure and anxiety, which could play a role in the urge to engage in self-injury. Additionally, it is apparent that Jenny is responding well to the school environment. Something is happening there that allows Jenny to cope differently with stress; thus, relationships with peers, coaches, and teachers, as well as engagement in other school supports, might be useful avenues to explore to support parent education.

Diversity issues

Several areas of diversity should be considered when working with Jenny. Her background is of multiple heritages (Asian, African American, and White). For a child this young, self-identifying and fitting in with peers become increasingly important. She may be seeking others who "look like" her to build her sense of self-concept (i.e., her relational experiences with individuals she identifies with can influence her perceptions of her abilities). Jenny is at a point in her life where she will begin to notice apparent differences typically specific to gender, race, and ethnicity/cultural beliefs. The need for Jenny to fit in and to be accepted by peers can influence how she engages at home (how she perceives her parents and herself in relation to them). The recent separation of her parents could create a divide for Jenny if she feels pressure to identify with any particular attributes she associates with her parents. Jenny's parents may also have different approaches to handling self-destructive behaviors and mental health issues due to cultural beliefs. There is often more of a stigma placed upon mental health problems and seeking counseling services in Asian and African American cultures. This, too, can create a sense of shame in Jenny and may be a source of conflict between her parents.

As Jenny is now nine years old, she is likely beginning to notice prepubescent changes. These pubescent changes can cause a greater focus on self in relation to peers and could influence her sense of self-worth. Her awareness of behavioral differences between boys and girls, and subsequent adult response to those differences, could also influence how Jenny engages in emotional communication and coping. The pressure to perform well can be linked to a variety of cultural expectations that intersect with gender normative expectations and racial identity. These are critical factors for teachers to be mindful of as they have Jenny in their classes. Often, teachers can unintentionally favor one gender or culture regarding educational expectations, performance, or support. Thus, parental values related to performance (chores, schoolwork, and sports) and Jenny's perceptions of those values/messages need to be further explored as potentially self-destructive coping mechanisms, as some may be protective, while others may be exacerbating problems.

Risk and protective factors

Jenny has several protective factors that are clinically significant. She appears to be very intelligent, as evidenced by her good grades. She does not show signs of active NSSI in school, which potentially indicates a lower stress experience at school and/or suggests that she has support for different coping strategies. Even if she is experiencing discomfort or anxiety at school, she can withhold the urge to engage in deliberate self-harm actively. Glenn and Klonsky (2010) note that urgency is the propensity to engage in impulsive actions or behaviors despite negative consequences, and this is the category that best describes the problems that self-injurers face. Jenny's ability to manage urgency is a protective factor and may indicate greater potential for a positive treatment outcome. Jenny has a coping technique or techniques that help her to manage stress, and this needs to be verbalized, encouraged, and integrated into treatment. In clinical samples, emotional dysregulation and self-derogation are related to family, school, and other interpersonal difficulties. Thus, emotional difficulties may foster and predict risk for NSSI in adolescence (Adrian et al., 2011). Before Jenny enters into adolescence, prevention practices (such as teaching coping and self-soothing strategies) could be useful in curbing this problem and avoiding the development of long-lasting, pervasive mental health issues.

Jenny appears to have a good relationship with her siblings, and her parents are potentially supportive of treatment. Parental support is critical in the treatment of NSSI. Previous research has indicated that there is a link between NSSI and family relational problems (Adrian et al., 2011; Martin et al., 2011). Since Jenny is actively engaging in NSSI and does not seem to be open to treatment, a focus on relationship building and motivational techniques will be important when working individually with her. Jenny insists her self-harm is "not a big deal," which indicates that she may not be ready to change. Recognition of healthy coping and encouragement of those patterns at home is particularly critical in helping Jenny to build positive experiences with other ways of managing stress and to be more motivated to change.

Case 1.2: Case of Sam

Sam is an 11-year-old, White male with a history of skin burning and interfering with wound healing (picking his scabs). Sam lives with his mother and has never had contact with his father. Sam's mother works long hours, which leaves Sam to walk to and from the school bus on his own, in addition to being home alone three to four hours a day before his mom gets home from work. During this time, Sam usually watches television and plays video games. He no longer spends time outdoors like he used to, and he sometimes stays up at night playing video games, getting less than five hours of sleep. Sam began burning his skin with pencil erasers when he was eight. His mother addressed it, but she didn't think too much of it and figured he would grow out of it. He seemed to do it when he was bored or when he appeared to be upset. Then, last year, after Sam was the target of some bullying at school, the burning behaviors seemed to escalate. Sam hid the bullying and burns for a long time. His mother noticed the new burns on his upper arms one day when they went to the community pool. Sam stated, "it's nothing, me and my friends thought the burn scars would be cool." He still denies that he burns himself, but his mom reports she's noticed more scabs on his forearms and has had to take him to the doctor for a few infections. When his mom discusses his picking and burns, he becomes enraged and punches holes in the walls, so she ultimately leaves him alone. Sam performs adequately in school and "wants to be left alone." He has a few friends and does not often engage in extracurricular activities. His grades are average, but slowly decreasing. He gets put in detention about once a week for his aggression and attitude toward his teacher and peers, but he doesn't seem to mind. When in detention, the proctor has noticed him picking at his skin, but she didn't think much of it and didn't say anything because he wasn't bothering anyone. His mother wants help, but she does not want to make the situation worse.

Developmental concerns

Sam is at an age where school and peers have become a priority in his life. Most of the time, when he is not at school, he is home alone. There is no one to connect with or to seek attention from. Sam is left to care for his own needs. Sam is also in the latter part of the industry v. inferiority stage in Erikson's developmental stages (Erikson, 1963). As mentioned earlier in this chapter, in this stage, children need support and encouragement from caregivers, parents, and teachers. Children seek a sense of accomplishment within this stage. Additionally, this is a very social age in development. Kids want to connect with others and seek out relationships from teachers and peers for support beyond their parents. Parents are no longer the only source of importance in their life. If children fail at achieving this milestone of development, they could be left feeling inadequate and inferior, as compared to those around them. These feelings can lead to problems with peers, isolation, competence, and self-esteem.

Sam does not appear to have mastered this stage of development. When Sam is at school, he does not have many social connections or friends. He is bullied by his peer group, which could be the cause of great stress, depression, anxiety, low self-esteem, further isolative behaviors, poor academic performance, and suicidal ideation/attempts (e.g., Bond et al., 2001; Klomek et al., 2007; Sourander et al., 2000). For some kids and teens, bullying within schools can contribute to self-harming behavior and further fuel the urge to self-injure, while for others, engagement in NSSI occurs as an initiation into a social group and as a means for peer acceptance. Sam is also in a stage of identity development. Self-harm is often not prioritized within school settings and planning curricula, and NSSI behaviors are often viewed as "bad behavior" where support is denied because it could escalate the behavior (Evans & Hurrell, 2016). Sam falls into these categories. He likely began his self-injurious behavior in order to deal with bullying and strong emotions, though he is getting some "positive" attention from the few friends he has who think his burn marks are "cool." Therefore, when faced with emotional turbulence, the NSSI behavior is reinforced by his situation. Additionally, Sam is at the pre- to early pubescent stage, which has the ability to affect his social world and cause anxiety. During this time, there is a surge of hormones and changes that take place in males and females. This can be overwhelming within the social and educational contexts. Children and teens who engage in NSSI as a method of coping are often left with few outlets at school when pubescent concerns clash with social and educational experiences.

Research with children also discusses a concept called *cold violence*, which is when children are ignored, neglected, shunned, or isolated by another child, person, or adult (Serra & Volpini, 2016). This *cold violence* seems to be what Sam unintentionally faces from adults around him. Sam's mother is absent for most of his day; his father is not in the picture; he is bullied at school; and his teachers and administrators seem to ignore the NSSI behavior or label him as "bad," as opposed to viewing it as a call for help and attention. In the industry v. inferiority stage of development, children need support and validation from those around them in order to feel successful and competent. His mother is too busy to give Sam what he needs, and she leaves him alone when he is engaging in NSSI behaviors (such as punching walls). She does not want to exacerbate or escalate the problem. Sam's mother is not intentionally trying to shun him, but she lacks the parenting skills to deal with the behavior. Leaving him alone does not provide Sam the support that he needs to cope. Family counseling would be beneficial for Sam to be able to express his needs to his mother and for his mother to receive some personal support and parental guidance. Sam's mother could also attend parenting classes and coaching to assist her in attaining a consistent parenting style that will help Sam.

Sam's school also does not appear to have a plan in place for working with NSSI or even recognizing NSSI behaviors. Sam needs support from teachers, but instead, he is faced with punishment and teachers who ignore him. Sam drastically lacks connection and support from all of those around him. A plan needs to be put in place with the school that allows them to be more vigilant in working with the NSSI behaviors that take place in school. Also, the plan should not be punishment based when Sam does engage in NSSI that is not threatening to others at school. More information on NSSI and working with schools is located in Chapter 9, but for now, Sam's mother needs to keep the lines of communication open with the school, navigate these challenging conversations, and come up with a safety-based plan if the school does see Sam engaging in NSSI while at school.

Additionally, Sam spends much of his alone time playing video games and watching television. As we know, there is a great deal of glamorizing violence that is displayed in video games and on television. There have been connections shown between aggression and television and video game usage among teens. The exposure to aggression can predispose and desensitize preschoolers, children, and teens to violence, aggressive thoughts, relationship aggression, and problematic parent and peer relationships (Coyne et al., 2017; Gentile et al., 2017; Johnson et al., 2002). The constant exposure to violence in various contexts is something that can set children up for failure developmentally.

Diversity issues

Sam is a White male. NSSI is consistently categorized and viewed as a behavior associated with females, more specifically, White females. Even though males are found to self-injure, the self-injury is often viewed as a form of aggression by teachers, parents, and professionals. Clinicians are also much less likely to assess for NSSI in males because of the gendered or stereotypical view of these behaviors (Whitlock et al., 2011). The self-injury itself also presents differently in males, which leads many males to misdiagnoses, and they are often viewed as aggressive or defiant because of the behavior (Healey et al., 2010). The displays in males are usually impulsive (like hitting or punching walls) when experiencing overwhelming or uncontrollable emotional experiences, and other less impulsive methods can often be a cry for help or social support and approval (Whitlock et al., 2011). When males are misdiagnosed, it results in ineffective or inappropriate treatment approaches. Typically, when this happens, the symptomology (anger) is treated as opposed to the etiology (or what caused the anger), which led to the feeling and NSSI behavior. Sam is at a critical age and approaching his teenage years. Sam will be facing many added pressures as he gets older. Without the appropriate interventions, his NSSI behaviors could progress, causing physical, emotional, or even legal consequences.

Additionally, Sam is from a lower socioeconomic status (SES) in that his family's income is just above the poverty line, and his mother has a high school education. He lives in a single-parent household and does not have easy access to community resources as transportation is unreliable, and he lives in an area with few public options. He has no male role models or figures he feels connected to. Being a male, as well as having a lack of males in his life for support, can increase suicidal ideation within the context of his perspective of his problems and increases the chances of NSSI eventually becoming more severe. Males take their own lives at nearly four times the rate of females. Suicide is also the third leading cause of death among persons aged 10–14, which is Sam's age group. Risk of suicide increases significantly within this age group. Additionally, from what is known about NSSI and Joiner's model, the Interpersonal-Psychological Theory of Suicide (IPTS; Joiner, 2005), the acquired capability for suicide stems from repeated exposure to habituated and painful events (e.g., self-injurious behavior). This will be discussed more in later chapters. Over time, the increase in the frequency of Sam's NSSI behavior is likely to become more severe if not properly diagnosed and treated.

For Sam, puberty can cause increased focus on himself in relation to his peers. He has few friends and seeks attention. Additionally, he thinks that the scars may "look cool." NSSI could be a way to gain this attention and to cope with this stress. Puberty, if not sooner, is often the stage when boys and girls begin to develop sexual feelings and attraction toward potential dating partners. Furthermore, this is a time that pre-teens and teens begin to contemplate their romantic orientation and attractions in a deeper way. For Sam, having few male or female peers could put more stress on him and cause him to isolate further. As a male, there is an ingrained stigma in American culture to be strong and not show emotions. For a pubescent male who lacks friends and social or romantic connections, isolation and displays of anger (NSSI) are the more acceptable methods of coping. This is a cultural expectation that often intersects with gender normative expression. With Sam having only maternal support, which is often limited due to his mother being the sole support for their family, he lacks other males in his life to provide comfort, validation, and/or guidance on how to deal with the male expectations that he faces in his social context.

Risk and protective factors

Sam's risk factors appear to be that he spends a great deal of time alone and has little adult supervision during the day. In addition to the lack of adult supervision, he has a lack of male figures in his life. Although Sam's mother is away for most of the day, it does seem as if she is supportive and doing the best that she can for Sam. Sam and his mother have a good relationship and do not report conflict between them. She wants to help Sam with this issue but seems uncertain how to meet this goal. She leaves him alone when he is actively engaging in NSSI behaviors, which further places Sam at risk. His school teachers seem uninterested in his NSSI behaviors and do not appear to understand that it is NSSI that he is engaging in. They do not give his NSSI behaviors attention and seek out punishment. He also does not give the impression that he has many friends, social supports, or emotional outlets. He seeks attention through scars that might appear "cool" to peers.

Additionally, Sam spends a great deal of his time watching television and playing video games. Considering Sam's current NSSI behaviors, exposure to violent video game content has the potential to exacerbate or worsen the NSSI behaviors. From what is known about NSSI, the longer someone engages in NSSI, the more frequent and severe the behaviors can become. This puts Sam at increased risk for suicidal ideation.

Sam appears to be cooperative. He has some peer relationships, which is important because he has not fully isolated himself. Sam enjoys the "praise" from his friends who think his NSSI burns are "cool." Even though we do not want Sam to hurt himself further to receive peer support and friendships, this shows us that he has a desire to belong and be accepted by his peers. He has not given up on friendships, which is positive. He does engage in some activities, which shows that Sam has motivation when he wants to put forth the effort. Sam is performing adequately in school and still has the desire to put energy into his grades so he does not fail.

TEXTBOX 1.1 REFLECTING ON GENDER

Sam and Jenny are only two years apart in age, but their NSSI presents very differently. The difference in their cultural backgrounds, parenting, and presentation of NSSI are evident. However, some may say their presentations of NSSI are different because of the role that gender plays. How do you see gender affecting the presentation in these two cases and their severity and methods of engagement in NSSI? What role do you feel that gender role stigma and norms play in these two case scenarios? A recent meta-analysis reported that differences in sex are minimal, if present at all (Swannell et al., 2014), while Bresin and Schoenleber's (2015) meta-analysis found females to be 1.5 times more likely to report NSSI engagement as compared to men. What factors do you think could be accounting for these differences when examining gender? How do these confounding factors affect your work clients who engage in NSSI but identify differently on the gender spectrum (i.e., male, female, genderfluid, or genderqueer)?

Conclusion

When working with Jenny and Sam, it will be critical to use evidence-based practices that will also address the diversity issues inherent in each case. The first step to work with both of these clients is realizing that the NSSI is occurring and connecting the patterns associated with the act. Clinicians working with young clients who self-injure should also consider the differences in the appearance of the behavior. Boys and men usually "act out" and do things that are visible and that could be considered aggressive. Girls and women typically "act in," and the behaviors are secretive and often hidden. Typically, for women, the behaviors are connected with depressive symptoms. The intersection of the client's gendered behaviors and the clinicians gender expectations have the potential to affect clinical conceptualization and treatment for that client. As the clinician, it is critical to consider the client's cultural and family values, especially when working with youth. Often, youth do not have the voice or ability to express themselves freely in opposition to cultural expectations that are thrust upon them. Children and adolescents usually fear the stigma of reporting and seeking help for self-harm. The way others view them directly affects their self-esteem and psyche at this critical time in development. Again, cultural context is not only crucial when assessing the self-injury, but also when considering the likeliness of help-seeking behaviors and the development of culture-specific interventions. More in-depth information about conceptualization will be discussed in Chapter 5 to help you, as the clinician, better understand why the self-injury is taking place, the purpose it serves, and which cultural contexts need consideration when conceptualizing the client and determining the most appropriate treatment plan.

Evidence-based practices with youth who engage in NSSI are limited due to the age of the clients when conducting randomized controlled trials. However, some treatments have revealed some effectiveness within small samples. When contemplating treatment for cases like Jenny and Sam, one of the main considerations is the developmental stage of the client and developmental appropriateness of the chosen intervention. For children, some techniques that are effective with adults, such as dialectical behavioral therapy (DBT), may not be effective in younger populations. Often, clients at this age may not have the ability to desire in-depth processing of emotions, thoughts, and feelings. This said, there are interventions that may be borrowed and adapted from various approaches. When working with children, play therapy, emotional regulation therapy, behavioral therapies (DBT, problem-solving therapies, and cognitive behavioral therapy), and family therapies have been shown to be effective. Play therapy helps to explore the child's world and inner thoughts in a fashion that is developmentally appropriate and fun for the child. Play therapy could be useful in connecting with Jenny and Sam. Cognitive-behavioral therapies could assist in assessing the motivation for the NSSI behaviors and processing the thought and emotional components related to the injury. DBT techniques that are developmentally appropriate show evidence of assisting with emotional regulation related to the self-injury. Family therapy will assist Jenny's and Sam's families to understand the function of the NSSI better and how they can change the dynamic in the family system to assist their children in treatment.

Clinical reflection

The *transtheoretical model of behavior change*, or *stages of change model*, provides five steps toward behavior change: precontemplation, contemplation, preparation for action, action, and maintenance. These stages are the way we typically assess a client's readiness to change a behavior and the first step in setting appropriate goals (see Table 1.2). However, younger children practicing self-injuring behaviors are less likely to be aware of why they are engaging in NSSI or how ready they are for change. You can attempt to gauge the child's readiness for change through the use of simple scaling questions, but often a child's age and developmental level will greatly affect change and their ability to process. Unless actively engaged in therapy, most children would be placed in the precontemplation stage, which is why examining their developmental level from a social cognitive theory perspective is also important. Social cognitive theory notes that change is determined through environmental, personal, and behavioral elements. All of these factors are highly interrelated and affect each other. We have to focus on the interactions of these factors in children because they are often not developmentally capable of processing this information. Additionally, they are less autonomous over the events that happen in their lives. They are dependent upon parents, caregivers, school environments, and other relationships that affect their behavior and the change process.

Table 1.2 Treatment goals

Client	*Short-term objective*	*Measure*	*Intervention*	*Stage of change and critical impacts*
Jenny	Create a safe atmosphere to identify the struggles at home and impact of parent-family relationships on self-injurious behaviors	Child Attachment Interview (CAI)	1. Child-centered play therapy to understand Jenny's worldview (e.g., sandtray) 2. Parenting skill-based training to learn how to set rules, discipline, and allow for choices.	Jenny and parents—precontemplation Impacts: Parents, school, coaches, peers
Sam	Increase awareness of how his lack of support from those around him is affecting his emotions and self-injurious behaviors	Children's Depression Rating Scale Revised (CDRS-R)	1. Family therapy to work toward a parent-child relationship. 2. Narrative therapy interventions, reauthoring, finding new meaning, and externalization to assist Sam in finding his strengths and gaining control.	Sam—precontemplation Mother—contemplation Impacts—mother, school, teachers, peers, and other relationships

Jenny's behavior at home versus in school appears to be very different. She seems to be very perfectionistic and a people pleaser. She is able to avoid injuring at school, which leads us to believe something is going on in her family environment that is causing the behavioral changes. Since parents and family are an integral part of the change process at this age, we would want to find out more about her attachment to her parents and her family environment. The Child Attachment Interview (CAI) is a narrative-based assessment that will help elicit Jenny's internal working model of attachment. The content of the CAI enables clinicians to evaluate the client's capacity for emotional regulation, and there are additional questions embedded about self-esteem, which is also relevant to attachment at this age. Since Jenny is nine years of age, play therapy would allow the therapist to fully explore Jenny's home life and how she views her world through activities such as sandtray therapy. Preteens are not only developing cognitive skills and seeking appraisals, but they are also developing creatively and moving in a direction that allows for abstract thought. Sandtray therapy would allow her to work through her issues and describe her world without being judged or feeling pressured. This is important, especially because Jenny has shown a perfectionistic quality, and we do not want her to feel the pressure of getting things right or pleasing us (as the therapist). The goal would be to allow Jenny to explore her worldview and put her home life in perspective, realizing that she is not at fault, nor can she control the outcome of situations between her parents. Rather, she can work through her feelings and come to an emotional understanding that will allow her to utilize the same coping skills she uses at school, at home. Jenny's parents have different attitudes about the seriousness of her NSSI, as evidenced by her mother's concern and her father's statement about "how much it really happens." Combining play therapy with family therapy and parental psychoeducation is critical to help all the socio-environmental factors and cultural impacts to come together toward the goal of behavioral change in Jenny.

Sam is at an age where support from those around him is critical. He has very few friends, his mother often leaves him home alone, and teachers at school do not want to be bothered with his NSSI behaviors (moreover, they provide punishment). Sam wants to "be left alone," and that is exactly what those around Sam do. Sam's bullying at school is affecting his self-esteem and self-image to the point that he is burning because it could "look cool" to peers. As a young male, Sam would need to be assessed for depression. He is currently displaying the following signs of depression that are commonly seen in young males: negative attitude, lack of interest, changes in sleep, decreased performance in school, anger outbursts, social isolation, and self-injurious behaviors. Utilizing the Children's Depression Rating Scale Revised, interviews can be conducted with Sam, his mother, and his teacher. Due to multiple raters, it is a comprehensive tool that is used to assess depression and to examine social withdrawal, sleep, fatigue, and suicidal ideation. It is important to understand if Sam is experiencing a mood disorder, such as depression or persistent depressive disorder so that the appropriate interventions can be set in place. Sam's primary goal is to stop self-injuring, but first, he needs to understand the function it has in his life. This does not only apply to Sam but to his mother as well. Family therapy will be needed to understand how patterns in the family are promoting Sam's self-injury. Currently, Sam feels invisible to all of those around him. It is critical that Sam participate in therapy with his mother, so he does not feel invisible, and they can both learn his triggers. Interventions, such as engaging in completing the "elementary-level safety plan" (see activity in Appendix B), would help Sam and his mother. This activity will help to understand Sam's needs and triggers while having something tangible to turn toward to assist with coping skills if someone is not present to help Sam when he wants to self-injure. Additionally, those things that he may be missing or where he has trouble identifying someone will help his mother get a clear picture of what he needs more of from her. Narrative therapy interventions would also benefit Sam (see Appendix A, psychotherapy.net for more information). Putting together his "story" and finding strength in the challenges that he overcomes at school with bullies will help build his confidence (see Appendix C for a storyboard activity). Externalizing the problems that he has at school will help Sam to realize he is not bad, but sometimes his behavior can be. Then he can learn that he has control over behaviors because those are external and can be changed. Deconstruction techniques will assist Sam in breaking down his problems into smaller ones that are easier to understand and address within his developmental level. Getting Sam's school counselor on board and involved with treatment will be critical, as Sam's school environment also plays a role in his self-injury.

REFERENCES

Adrian, M., Zeman, J., Erdley, C., Lisa, L., & Sim, L. (2011). Emotional dysregulation and interpersonal difficulties as risk factors for nonsuicidal self-injury in adolescent girls. *Journal of Abnormal Child Psychology*, 39(3), 389–400. doi:10.1007/s10802-010-9465-3

Andover, M.S., Morris, B.W., Wren, A., & Bruzzese, M.E. (2012). The co-occurrence of non-suicidal self-injury and attempted suicide among adolescents: Distinguishing risk factors and psychosocial correlates. *Child and Adolescent Psychiatry and Mental Health*, 6(1), 11. doi:10.1186/1753-2000-6-11

Baetens, I., Claes, L., Hasking, P., Smits, D., Grietens, H., Onghena, P., & Martin, G. (2015). The relationship between caregivers' expressed emotions and non-suicidal self-injury: The mediating roles of self-criticism and depression. *Journal of Child and Family Studies*, 24(2), 491–498. doi:10.1007/s10826-013-9861-8

Barrocas, A.L., Hankin, B.L., Young, J.F., & Abela, J.R. (2012). Rates of nonsuicidal self-injury in youth: Age, sex, and behavioral methods in a community sample. *Pediatrics*, 130(1), 39–45. doi:10.1542/peds.2011-2094

Bond, L., Carlin, J.B., Thomas, L., Rubin, K., & Patton, G. (2001). Does bullying cause emotional problems? A prospective study of young teenagers. *British Medical Journal*, 323(7311), 480–484. doi:10.1136/bmj.323.7311.480

Bresin, K., & Schoenleber, M. (2015). Gender differences in the prevalence of nonsuicidal self-injury: A meta-analysis. *Clinical Psychology Review*, 38, 55–64. doi:10.1016/j.cpr.2015.02.009

Centers for Disease Control and Prevention (CDC). (2017). 10 Leading causes of death by age group, United States – 2017. Retrieved from https://www.cdc.gov/injury/images/lc-charts/leading_causes_of_death_by_age_group_2017_1100w850h.jpg

Coyne, S.M., Stockdale, L., Linder, J.R., Nelson, D.A., Collier, K.M., & Essig, L.W. (2017). Pow! Boom! Kablam! Effects of viewing superhero programs on aggressive, prosocial, and defending behaviors in preschool children. *Journal of Abnormal Child Psychology*, 45, 1523–1535. doi:10.1007/s10802-016-0253-6

Erikson, E. (1963). *Childhood and Society* (2nd ed., rev. and enl.). New York, NY: Norton.

Evans, R., & Hurrell, C. (2016). The role of schools in children and young people's self-harm and suicide: Systematic review and meta-ethnography of qualitative research. *BMC Public Health*, 16(1), 401. doi:10.1186/s12889-016-3065-2

Fliege, H., Lee, J.R., Grimm, A., & Klapp, B.F. (2009). Risk factors and correlates of deliberate self-harm behavior: A systematic review. *Journal of Psychosomatic Research*, 66, 477–493. doi:10.1016/j.jpsychores.2008.10.013

Gentile, D.A., Bender, P.K., & Anderson, C.A. (2017). Violent video game effects on salivary cortisol, arousal, and aggressive thoughts in children. *Computers in Human Behavior*, 70, 39–43. doi:10.1016/j.chb.2016.12.045

Glenn, C.R., & Klonsky, E.D. (2010). A multimethod analysis of impulsivity in nonsuicidal self-injury. *Personality Disorders: Theory, Research, and Treatment*, 1(1), 67. doi:10.1037/a0017427

Healey, A., Trepal, H., & Emelianchik-Key, K. (2010). Nonsuicidal self-injury: Examining the relationship between diagnosis and gender. *Journal of Mental Health Counseling*, 32(4), 324–341. doi:10.17744/mehc.32.4.366740506r458202

Hughes, D. (2004). An attachment-based treatment of maltreated children and young people. *Attachment and Human Development*, 6, 263–278. doi:10.1080/14616730412331281539

Johnson, J.G., Cohen, P., Smailes, E.M., Kasen, S., & Brook, J.S. (2002). Television viewing and aggressive behavior during adolescence and adulthood. *Science*, 295, 2468–2471. doi:10.1126/science.1062929

Joiner, Jr., T.E. (2005). *Why People Die by Suicide*. Cambridge, MA: Harvard University Press.

Kaess, M., Parzer, P., Mattern, M., Plener, P.L., Bifulco, A., Resch, F., & Brunner, R. (2013). Adverse childhood experiences and their impact on frequency, severity, and the individual function of nonsuicidal self-injury in youth. *Psychiatry Research*, 206(2–3), 265–272. doi:10.1016/j.psychres.2012.10.012

Kelada, L., Whitlock, J., Hasking, P., & Melvin, G. (2016). Parents' experiences of nonsuicidal self-injury among adolescents and young adults. *Journal of Child and Family Studies*, 25(11), 3403–3416. doi:10.1007/s10826-016-0496-4

Klomek, A.B., Marrocco, F., Kleinman, M., Schonfeld, I.S., & Gould, M.S. (2007). Bullying, depression, and suicidality in adolescents. *Journal of the American Academy of Child Psychology*, 46, 40–49. doi:10.1097/01.chi.0000242237.84925.18

Klonsky, E.D. (2007). The functions of deliberate self-injury: A review of the evidence. *Clinical Psychology Review*, 27(2), 226–239. doi:10.1016/j.cpr.2006.08.002

Lamela, D., Figueiredo, B., Bastos, A., & Feinberg, M. (2016). Typologies of post-divorce coparenting and parental well-being, parenting quality and children's psychological adjustment. *Child Psychiatry and Human Development*, 47(5), 716–728. doi:10.1007/s10578-015-0604-5

Martin, J., Bureau, J.F., Cloutier, P., & Lafontaine, M.F. (2011). A comparison of invalidating family environment characteristics between university students engaging in self-injurious thoughts and actions and non-self-injuring university student. *Journal of Youth and Adolescence*, 40(11), 1477–1488. doi:10.1007/s10964-011-9643-9

Muehlenkamp, J.J., Claes, L., Havertape, L., & Plener, P.L. (2012). International prevalence of adolescent non-suicidal self-injury and deliberate self-harm. *Child and Adolescent Psychiatry and Mental Health*, 6(1), 10. doi:10.1186/1753-2000-6-10

Piaget, J. (1976). Piaget's theory. In *Piaget and His School* (pp. 11–23). Springer, Berlin, Heidelberg. doi:10.1007/978-3-642-46323-5_2

Serra, O., & Volpini, L. (2016). Considerations about cold violence. *Caderno CRH*, 29(76), 119–132. doi:10.1590/s0103-49792016000100008

Sourander, A., Helstelä, L., Helenius, H., & Piha, J. (2000). Persistence of bullying from childhood to adolescence—a longitudinal 8-year follow-up study. *Child Abuse & Neglect*, 24(7), 873–881. doi:10.1016/s0145-2134(00)00146-0

Swannell, S.V., Martin, G.E., Page, A., Hasking, P., & St John, N.J. (2014). Prevalence of non-suicidal self-injury in nonclinical samples: Systemic review, meta-analysis and meta-regression. *Suicide and Life-Threatening Behavior*, 44(3), 273–303. doi:10.1111/sltb.12070

Whitlock, J., Muehlenkamp, J., Purington, A., Eckenrode, J., Barreira, P., Baral Abrams, G., … & Knox, K. (2011). Nonsuicidal self-injury in a college population: General trends and sex differences. *Journal of American College Health*, 59, 691–698. doi:10.1080/07448481.2010.529626

2 Non-suicidal self-injury in adolescents and young adults

Amanda La Guardia

As previously noted, self-directed violence in the form of non-suicidal self-injury is of growing concern for clinicians working with youth, mostly due to the behavior's link to suicidal ideation and attempt behaviors. As a reminder, suicide is the second leading cause of death for children and young adults aged 10–34 (CDC, 2016). NSSI has been noted as a pervasive issue among the adolescent population, with prevalence rates in psychiatric adolescent samples as high as 60% for one occurrence and around 50% for repeat occurrences over a 12-month period (Kaess et al., 2013). A recent analysis of the research on non-clinical youth found NSSI to be occurring in 17.2% of adolescents and 13.4% of young adults (Swanell et al., 2014). NSSI is typically thought to be a female issue. Thus, participants in research tend to be predominantly young adult females (Marchetto, 2006). Additionally, self-injury among males may not be clinically conceptualized in the same way as for female self-injurers (Healey et al., 2010). However, NSSI is an issue that affects both males and females at similar rates and is prevalent across cultures within Western societies.

Here we present three different client cases to serve as examples for the conceptualization and treatment of NSSI in adolescent and young adult populations.

We delineate clinical decision-making procedures about treatment progression and review developmentally and culturally oriented risk and protective factors that pertain to each case. This information will also be further detailed in Part II of this book.

Case 2.1: Case of Emma

The case of Emma will focus on systemic approaches that include peer group counseling, individual counseling, and family counseling interventions as a way to highlight preferred and evidenced-based methods for addressing the behavior.

Emma is a 17-year-old Latina who has been having difficulties at home and school. She has been living with her grandmother since the age of 10 after being removed from her mother's home. She was placed with her fraternal grandmother after reports of sexual abuse by her 13-year-old biological brother and 16-year-old stepbrother. Her grandmother reports that the client has been very irritable and isolating herself from the family for the past two years, and she worries about depression since Emma's father died by suicide when Emma was seven. Before age 15, it was reported that the client had frequent nightmares and was relatively shy, but she did not have any overtly disruptive behavioral problems. Emma was recently hospitalized for cutting herself on the forearm with a razor in her high school bathroom. Her grandmother stated that she had previously noticed burn marks on the client's arms. Emma has refused to do work in school or follow the instructions given by her teachers. She frequently goes to the school nurse during the day for headaches, and her grades have been steadily dropping since the beginning of the school year. Since the start of the school year, she has also been in two physical fights with other students. At home, Emma spends most of her time in her room listening to music and refuses to eat dinner with her grandmother. She becomes argumentative when asked to do chores or contribute to household duties. Emma's grandmother states that when she noticed the burn marks, she began talking with Emma nightly, but her grandmother reports that most of the conversation revolved around Emma's desire to leave school and her annoyance at completing household chores. Emma was hospitalized a year prior for suicidal ideation.

Upon initially meeting with Emma, you ask her about the recent hospitalization. She tells you that she burned herself with ice and salt while in treatment and was upset when the staff would not let her use implements that would result in self-injury. Emma refuses to talk about her family and instead focuses the discussion around self-injury. She states that it made her feel better, but she cannot articulate how she felt when she would self-injure or why it made her feel better. She indicates that she has one close friend and informs the counselor that they often hang out together and listen to music while smoking and burn themselves with their cigarettes. Emma asserts that she has no desire to change her self-injury: "It helps, and people just need to accept it and stop freaking out about it." Emma's grandmother is interested in being involved in treatment but notes that her husband is very busy with his job and is rarely able to participate in Emma's treatment.

Developmental perspective

Emma is in a psychosocial stage associated with identity development, which is characterized by role identification ("How do I fit in?") and the development of the ability to accept others, even when there are differences between them. Trauma can sometimes limit psychosocial development during the stage at which it occurred, which for Emma is between the ages of 7 and 10, at the point of her father's suicide and her subsequent sexual abuse. During this point in Emma's maturation, she was focusing on fostering relationships with her peers, who would be a major source of her self-esteem. She would have needed acceptance and affirmation to develop a sense of competence, with a balance between failure and achievement. This stage would have occurred just before Emma's current, age-specific stage, and thus both could play a role in her perception of current issues. In terms of cognitive development, Emma experienced significant trauma during her concrete operational stage. This is when children learn that everyone has their thoughts and feelings, and those thoughts and feelings could be different from their own. During this time, logic and reasoning also begin to develop, encouraging deeper understanding and awareness of patterns. Emma is currently in a formal operational stage of development, allowing her to consider multiple possibilities and solutions along with abstract concepts, such as equity and justice. Due to Emma's trauma, she may have a limited ability to think abstractly, wavering between formal and concrete operations.

Research indicates that when sexual abuse occurs during certain sensitive periods in development, lasting effects on brain structure and function may result (but no consistent evidence indicates these changes are irreversible). For Emma, her abuse occurred during one of these sensitive periods, potentially reducing cortex gray matter volume, which is linked to social cognition and functional organization (namely, her ability to differentiate her perspective and needs from others or predict the behavior of others). Further, her ability to monitor her actions internally in relation to a situational context may have been dampened (Baker et al., 2013; Kahn et al., 2015). It is likely that Emma is experiencing or has experienced symptoms associated with post-traumatic stress. Due to the timing of the suicide of her father, her sexual abuse, and her transition into care, she may associate certain peer behaviors with abuse; thus, she may struggle to predict the actions (safe or unsafe) of others and may still blame herself for her adverse experiences. Her self-injury could serve as a form of self-punishment. Therefore, assessing her level of insight, impulsivity, and perspective of self in regard to others might be beneficial in developing useful interventions designed to help Emma examine her needs and invest in exploring new coping strategies.

Diversity issues

Emma identifies as Latina. While there are common values associated with individuals from Latin cultures, Emma's family may not ascribe to these values or may not attend to them rigidly. Thus, an exploration of family expectations, values, and stories might be useful in the process of exploring Emma's self-perception. Emma's grandmother might also be a good resource for understanding the family's history and cultural traditions, as grandparents in Hispanic cultures may view their role as being an emissary of the culture, religion, and language of the family. Typically, Latin or Hispanic families prefer to rely on the family to solve problems, related to a concept known as *familism* (Zayas et al., 2009). This family is seeking help from external resources. Given the family is soliciting help from outside of the family, Emma may be experiencing culture-related stressors (see Cervantes et al., 2014). It will be important to explore how the family is characterizing counseling and how this influences Emma's perspective (e.g., the belief that she does not need help, and that people, perhaps her grandparents, need to be more accepting of her self-injury). Emma may feel like a burden on her grandparents and may not want them to worry, which could influence the way she communicates with them, potentially exacerbating the issue if she does not feel able to rely on her grandparents for emotional support.

Risk and protective factors

Emma has one close friend with whom she spends time, indicating that she can develop and maintain relationships with peers. She likely also cares about her grandparents and may desire their approval or to protect them from her pain. Emma has also shown that she can find her resources to manage her emotional struggles. While self-injury is not a healthy coping strategy, she has found something that is working for her. However, it will be important to assess how Emma's friendship is emotionally supportive and how it may be contributing to her self-injurious behaviors. Many times, adolescents who self-injure also have a friend who does. Their friendship could include self-injury, which may make it more difficult for Emma to stop. If this friend is Emma's sole source for emotional support, Emma may fear damaging the relationship if she were to stop self-injuring.

Treatment will need to begin with the development of motivation and insight, and an assessment of family values, needs, and Emma's sense of belongingness and self-efficacy with regard to peer relationships. Initial goals may focus on emotional awareness, communication skill development, and distress tolerance. Once Emma invests in changing her self-injurious behaviors, she may be more receptive to family and group counseling, which would increase the likelihood of their success. For more information on assessment and processing of readiness for treatment of self-injury, see Cornell University's *Self-Injury and Recovery Research and Resources* (2019).

Case 2.2: Case of Rick

Rick frequently and intentionally engages in self-burning using an eraser. He also instigates physical altercations at school, during which he is physically hurt. He deals with frustrations at home by punching walls and engages in scarification. We address the intersections of cultural experience and support as a function of case presentation.

Rick is a 14-year-old Black male who lives with his father and younger brother. His mother lost her parental rights when Rick was four after she was incarcerated on drug-related charges and child neglect. Over the last year, Rick frequently instigates physical altercations at school, which tend to result in Rick requiring medical attention. His father believes the fights happen on days when Rick seems upset but thinks the aggression is "a boy thing" and would like to redirect it into a sport; however, Rick has no interest in playing sports. Rick always initiates the altercations (usually in the lunchroom or when school lets out). He is often left with physical injuries and appears calm when removed from the situation by school faculty or staff. Rick is not engaged in academics and is barely passing his classes. Rick has a few friends whom his father considers to be "bad influences." However, his father seems to like Rick's girlfriend, who is a senior in the same high school. He thinks the relationship might be good for him and says he is proud that his son is attracting female attention, noting that Rick's girlfriend is attractive.

His father is not overly concerned about the fighting and wants a counselor to help get Rick interested in sports and ensure he graduates from high school. He believes Rick would get the "discipline he needs" from being part of a sports team and will learn "what it takes to do well in life." Rick's grandmother is very involved with Rick and his brother and reports she is concerned over the age difference in Rick's intimate relationship and thinks the girlfriend might be using drugs. She also reports that Rick seems to be burning designs into his skin and does not attend church with her and his younger brother much anymore. Rick will not contribute to the household and will punch holes in walls. He refuses to communicate with his father or grandmother when they attempt to discipline him. His grandmother says he is "agreeable" but "will not talk" and typically just walks out of the house during any incidents of disagreement. Rick has had recent psychological and educational testing through his school due to ongoing academic and behavioral concerns. As a result, he was diagnosed with oppositional defiance disorder and attention deficit disorder (ADD). During an individual education planning (IEP) meeting, which occurs in response to identified academic and/or behavioral needs, the school psychologist offered a referral to the family for Rick to see a psychiatrist for medication management of his symptoms. However, Rick's father has not followed up on the referral because he does not want his son "drugged." Rick's grandmother believes her son needs to be more active in Rick's life and that Rick needs to return to church. She "appreciates" any help, but she believes counseling should focus on church and family. Rick seems ambivalent about spending more time at church, but he does state that he is interested in finding other ways to manage his feelings that do not include a physical response (i.e., fighting and hitting walls), as these actions seem to, in his words, "cause more trouble than it's worth." Rick believes his relationship with his girlfriend is "rocky" but says "she needs me right now" so wants to "be there for her." He states that his friends keep him "grounded" and that they'll be there for each other "for life," and this helps him to feel good when he's feeling "down about stuff."

Developmental perspective

Rick has recently begun his adolescence and transitioned to high school, where he is struggling socially and academically. It would be appropriate to explore any changes in Rick's friend group and how he perceives his role within that group, as well as his perception of his intimate partnership. Peer relationships are extremely important in adolescent identity development. Additionally, Rick may be seeking approval from adults he perceives as an ideal representation of his personal developmental goals. While it may appear that this person might not be Rick's father given the defiance at home, Rick could still be feeling a need for his father's approval (but may feel discouraged about receiving it). In exploring identity development, it might be helpful for Rick to think about the values he has learned from his family (e.g., father and grandmother) and how those values influence his self-perception. What kind of person does he think he is now? What kind of adult does he hope to become? At this point in his life, Rick is potentially moving away from childhood beliefs about himself and others and forming new ideas about his place in the world, within his family, in intimate relationships, and his sense of self-efficacy. This is a lot for anyone to think about and naturally leads to emotional challenges typical of adolescents. However, if Rick does not feel a strong sense of support from caregivers, he may feel alone in this developmental process and may not have a space to express his concerns about self or others. His re-evaluation of identity and his place in the world may be influencing changes in church attendance as well as his desire to communicate his feelings to his grandmother.

Diversity issues

Rick's father is very focused on rigid ideals of masculinity (i.e., lack of concern over fighting and attractiveness of his girlfriend) and academic achievement (i.e., a desire he graduate from high school). The values communicated to Rick regarding his beliefs about a man's role in a relationship, with peers, and at home could influence how Rick approaches those areas of his life. Those stated values may also affect Rick's willingness to engage in discussion about them with his father. If a conflict exists between his father's expectations and his own experiences, heightened emotional distress could result. This is indicated by Rick's defiant behavior toward his father and grandmother and may potentially be affecting his behavior toward authority figures at school. However, Rick may also believe that he should be "strong" (which typically implies suppression of emotions in men). He may use fighting as a perceived socially acceptable way to express his feelings but also to stop or regulate them. Exploring his father's desire to have Rick get involved in sports and his grandmother's interest in re-engaging him with "church and family" may assist a counselor in aligning therapeutic goals with family values. In order to determine how cultural and family values may be influencing family relationships and Rick's interest in and ability to communicate his issues with adults and peers, it would be useful to broach the topic of masculinity in counseling. Rather than making cultural assumptions, allow Rick to discuss how he perceives expectations of masculinity from his father and grandmother versus how he thinks of his role with his friends and in his intimate relationship. These messages could be influencing his process of emotional expression, which may be linked to his engagement in self-injurious behaviors, as evidenced by his use of gender-appropriate expressions of injury (i.e., fighting and scarification). For more on minority issues and non-suicidal self-injury, see Chesin et al. (2013).

Risk and protective factors

Rick's grandmother seems to be invested in his family and community relationships (e.g., father-son relationship and faith community), while Rick's father is invested in his appearance of success (e.g., peer relationships, girlfriend, and academic completion). Discussing the family's perspectives on their strengths can assist the clinician in identifying risk and protective factors relevant to the functioning of the family and Rick's behaviors. In numerous research studies over the past decade, family dysfunction and perceived dysfunction have been associated with suicidal behaviors. In a study of self-injurers, non-injurers, and past self-injures, Hack and Graham (2018) indicate that perceived criticism from family members, experiences of shame, and psychological distress contributed to and predicted self-injurious behaviors, whereas emotional involvement of the family protected individuals from self-injury. With regard to parenting, Victor et al. (2019) suggested that parental punishment, low parental monitoring, and poor attachment are potentially related to adolescent self-injurious behaviors, while positive parenting (e.g., parent availability and sensitivity) seemed to protect adolescents from the onset of self-injury. Although this research was completed with a female sample population, the findings indicate that parent relationships may be an important area of focus for clinicians. Parenting has been a particular focus for risky behaviors in youth; thus, it is no surprise that addressing it may be important for youth engaging in self-injury. Youth need to feel a meaningful sense of support and connection within their family. Simple inclusion is not enough to protect from emotional distress.

Social contagion is a real concern when working with adolescent clients, as peer support has been demonstrated to have a strong relationship with self-injurious behaviors. Victor et al. (2019) also found that peer victimization and poor social self-worth were uniquely related to the onset of non-suicidal self-injury. Social contagion theory includes assertive relations (predispositional attitudes and beliefs lead to group attraction), direct imitation (e.g., peer influence), and indirect imitation (e.g., media influence). The majority of youth who self-injure tend to have a friend who also engages in the behavior. NSSI is influenced by social will, meaning it is largely socially constructed. How individual youth choose to engage in and communicate with others about self-injury is thus influenced by social context as well as psychological factors. Self-esteem can be a protective process, allowing for self-preservation and resiliency within environments that may influence the adoption and maintenance of risky or self-destructive behaviors.

TEXTBOX 2.1 REFLECTING ON CULTURE AND RACE

Recent research indicates prevalence rates for NSSI among adolescents and youth are higher for White and Asian groups (see Chesin et al., 2013) in the United States. General prevalence rates among non-White youth are similar to those of White youth. While Chesin's study found no protective link between NSSI and ethnic identity, it did suggest that interfamilial differences in acculturation might play a role in the use of NSSI more so than individual internal conflict regarding race and culture. Chesin's study did find a protective trend for Hispanic ethnicity, while other studies have found a potential protective trend for African American ethnicity in youth.

Given this, how will you explore the potential cultural strengths Hispanic and African American youth might bring to treatment when working to change NSSI behaviors? How could cultural protective factors influence the development of treatment goals and interventions?

Case 2.3: Case of Charlotte

The case of Charlotte focuses on work with a White, bisexual, non-binary female attending university and struggling with the coming-out process. We explore the intersections of gender expectations and identity development concerning NSSI through individual treatment modalities in a higher education setting.

Charlotte is a White, bisexual non-binary female, who is 19 years old. She has been cutting, burning, and scratching since the age of 15. She was molested by her maternal grandfather from the ages of six to nine but believed it could have been longer; she does not remember. She has a healthy relationship with her mother, but still struggles with the fact that her abuse happened for so long. Her mother walked in on the abuse and quickly cut off the relationship with her grandfather, but she refused to press charges. Charlotte's grandfather died two years later, and Charlotte reports that she never received treatment for her abuse. Charlotte's biological father left the family when she was three years old, which is when her grandfather stepped in to help. Charlotte's grandmother has Alzheimer's disease; she has been in an inpatient assisted-living facility since Charlotte was five years of age. Charlotte's mom remarried when she was eight years old and then had another baby. Her stepfather is "very pleasant," and they are both on "good terms." Her stepfather was strict with Charlotte and her brother as they grew up, so she had very little social life and was hardly ever allowed to date or interact with boys; however, she reports that this rarely ever bothered her. Charlotte frequently would engage in playing sports and was sometimes viewed as a tomboy, though she also liked to spend time with her mom and would do things that were "feminine" in nature (e.g., shopping for clothes and going to the spa) to please her mother. Around the age of 15, Charlotte started having feelings for her female best friend, and eventually, the two became intimate with one another. Charlotte struggled with this development, and then ended the relationship about one year after they began being intimate. She was terrified her stepfather or mother would find out. At the time of the relationship, she wondered if she was a lesbian and often considered what that meant for her family relationships. Her stepfather is highly regarded in her community, so Charlotte often wonders if something must be wrong with her since everyone is so approving of him. Charlotte began to feel depressed and withdrew from people socially. Around the age of 18, Charlotte's mom took her to a therapist. This was shortly before she went off to college. Charlotte admitted to self-injuring and explained to the therapist how she has never felt comfortable in her skin. Charlotte worked with the therapist for three months and felt like she had gotten better. She rarely engaged in self-injury over the next six months. At present, Charlotte is in college, taking classes full-time, and living on her own. She has started to self-injure again and has been restricting her food intake. She is also involved in a relationship with another female student that is getting serious. Charlotte is struggling with telling her mother and stepfather about the relationship. Last week, Charlotte's mother said they are coming for a visit next month. Later that day, Charlotte cut herself so deeply that she needed medical attention. The university physician has required her to come and see you. Charlotte insists it was an accident and did not realize how deeply she cut. You have six sessions with Charlotte due to policy restrictions for yearly student counseling visits. The school is requiring Charlotte to attend counseling since she engaged in this self-injurious act on campus and her dorm. Her RA was the one that brought her to the physician. She reports being active in the gay-straight alliance on campus and feels supported by staff at the LGBT center. Charlotte is open to counseling and states that she "does not want to self-injure," but she feels like it is the only method "that works" reliably when she is overwhelmed.

Developmental perspective

Identity development can be a fluid process that includes intersections between the development of a person's self-concept, connections to peer groups and community, and family relationships. Sexual orientation identity process models, like the one discussed by D'Augelli (1994), indicate that identity can be fixed and fluid, depending on both environmental and biological factors. (See Bilodeau & Renn, 2005, for a review of the process, stage, and other models associated with gender and orientation identity development within the context of university-based supports and policy.) Facilitating a discussion with Charlotte about her self-concept in relation to her perceptions of her parent's values and beliefs may assist with her identify conflict, which seems to be tied to her self-injurious behaviors. Exploring her self-concept about her strengths and challenges can be addressed through narrative exposure therapy (NET), which is a culturally inclusive, conditionally evidenced process for the treatment of trauma and symptoms associated with trauma experience. NET assists clients in developing a healthy perspective of personal identity within the context of their life experiences.

Because Charlotte's sexual abuse occurred during a point in her development where she would have been building a sense of self-confidence, this area of her self-concept may be affected by the abuse, which would have then influenced the development of her sense of self. As Charlotte was moving through a concrete operational stage of cognitive development, she may have attributed her pattern of abuse to herself, which is a common result of childhood sexual abuse experience. Currently, Charlotte is struggling with the psychosocial stage of intimacy versus isolation, which might be particularly difficult for her given that she may have fear associated with intimacy on multiple levels (i.e., she may blame problems in the relationship on herself, she may believe her feelings for women are not acceptable or won't be accepted by her family, etc.). Any treatment approach implemented must be mindful of Charlotte's developmental challenges as well as her prior developmental experiences.

Diversity issues

In numerous studies published in the last decade, LGBTQ identification has been associated with increased incidence of self-injury and suicide. Charlotte identifies as bisexual, which has been associated with heightened levels of self-injury, beyond those reporting to be exclusively gay/lesbian or straight (Benau et al., 2017). While parental disclosure of sexual orientation has generally been demonstrated to reduce lifetime NSSI, when parental control occurs in conjunction with disclosure, it has been demonstrated to increase lifetime NSSI for those who identify as bisexual or mixed orientation. Thus, parental disclosure should not be a therapeutic goal; rather, the development of healthy parental communication and identity confidence is a more effective approach, as it will create space for Charlotte to decide when and if she wants to disclose her sexual orientation to her parents. Additionally, Charlotte identifies as non-binary, and thus, she may feel that she must perform her biologically perceived gender around her parents, further complicating her relationship with them. Hiding these parts of her identity can also cause high levels of minority-related stress, which is also a risk factor for frequent and severe NSSI.

Risk and protective factors

Charlotte appears to have concerns with being open about her gender and sexual identity with her family. However, she seems to question these concerns as they relate to her self-concept. Helping Charlotte to evaluate her thoughts and feelings in a way that values both identities may assist her in recognizing and affirming her internal appraisal process rather than engaging in self-criticism. Charlotte is involved in a healthy intimate relationship, which may serve as strong peer support for her. Evaluating how Charlotte's partner could become involved in her treatment might assist in preventing future self-injury, as social connectedness has been demonstrated to be a protective factor for sexual minority youth (Taliaferro & Muehlenkamp, 2017). Meyer's minority stress model may serve to be a useful way to conceptualize of the risks and protective factors facing sexual minority individuals specific to experiences of discrimination and victimization. While Charlotte reports a good relationship with both her stepfather and mother, the messages they provide related to sexual orientation and gender expression may have created an atmosphere in which Charlotte felt her identity would not be and is not valued. Thus, supports within her educational and peer environment will serve as a strong foundation for psychological safety, as Charlotte works to address factors contributing to her self-injury. Charlotte will need to work through her past sexual abuse from her grandfather, which is a strong risk factor for lifetime NSSI. Her grandmother has Alzheimer's, but even so, it may assist Charlotte to get closure with her grandmother now and to address the abuse by her grandfather, so she can begin to cope with it as opposed to burying it. Her past abuse history is also a risk factor for her eating disordered behavior. NSSI and eating disorders often co-exist in clients. There is a high prevalence of shame, body dissatisfaction, impulsivity, cognitive distortions, emotional avoidance, and a lack of self-esteem in those who engage in both behaviors. It is likely that her past abuse, gender minority stress, and the transition into college are all weighing on her eating disordered behaviors and her self-injury. She no longer has the protective factor of her parents, who may have kept her from engaging in disordered eating behaviors. Seeking out more support resources on campus, like nutritional support services and peer support groups, could assist with getting her eating habits back on track. Her partner could also serve as a source of support and protective factors, as she attempts to organize her routine to encompass healthy eating habits.

TEXTBOX 2.2 REFLECTING ON SEXUAL MINORITY STATUS AND NSSI

According to Taliaferro and Muehlenkamp (2017), "Bisexual youth might face unique challenges during adolescence associated with their sexual orientation, such as lack of acceptance by heterosexual as well as homosexual peers, thus, experiencing less connectedness within the lesbian, gay, bisexual, transgender, and queer (LGBTQ) community" (p. 718). Reports indicate the sexual minority youth are two to four times more likely to attempt suicide over their lifetime than non-sexual minority youth.

Knowing this and some of the risk and protective factors associated with non-suicidal self-injury, how might you participate in your health community to advocate for sexual minority youth? For more on public health advocacy as it relates to mental health, please visit the World Health Organization's paper on "Advocacy for Mental Health" (visit: https://www.who.int/mental_health/policy/services/1_advocacy_WEB_07.pdf).

Conclusion

Multiple treatment protocols have demonstrated effectiveness in working with self-injurious youth and adults. Primarily, motivational interviewing (to build investment in change), dialectical behavioral therapies, emotional regulation group therapy, manualized cognitive behavior therapies, and some SSRIs have all been shown to reduce the frequency of self-injurious behaviors as well as overall self-harm in randomized controlled trials (Turner et al., 2014). Family counseling is also helpful, once a youth is ready to invest in stopping self-injurious behavior. Having a caregiver present to encourage and support new coping methods and practice healthy communication strategies is important for lasting change. May your pride never exceed your shine, nor your humility dull it. Learning to recognize strengths and highlight them within relationships is an essential and healthy way to communicate needs. Sometimes individuals who self-injure struggle with valuing themselves and thus they can devalue their needs in relation to others or attempt to feel valuable by trying to be perceived as better than others are. These states may present as a swing, both occurring at different times. Health communication techniques can assist these individuals in balancing that swing.

There is evidence that reinforcement plays a role in supporting NSSI behaviors in four ways. The first two are intrapersonal in nature, meaning they address internal experience. Intrapersonal negative reinforcement is a mechanism that results in the reduction of overwhelming emotions like anger or, most typically, anxiety. The second is intrapersonal positive reinforcement that results in relief of numbness or internal emptiness/dissonance. Both of these mechanisms indicate issues with emotional dysregulation. These two behavioral reinforcements have also been associated with increased self-injury severity and suicide risk (Brausch & Muehlenkamp, 2018). The final two functions of self-injury are interpersonal in nature. Interpersonal negative reinforcement occurs when individuals engage in self-injury to reduce perceived victimization (e.g., to stop a bullying incident), and positive interpersonal reinforcement occurs when the individual is attempting to get attention or gain emotional support from peers. The functions have been linked to lower rates of lifetime NSSI, and these individuals are also less likely to engage in suicidal behaviors than those using self-injury to address intrapersonal functions (Brausch & Muehlenkamp, 2018).

Research conducted by Burke et al. (2018) on latent class factors influencing NSSI in youth indicates that there is a specific group of factors influencing engagement in NSSI over time. Late adolescents who were in a moderate negative coping class reported above-average levels of negative affect, lower positive affect, brooding, and reflection, coupled with below-average levels of positive affect and positive rumination. These adolescents were more likely to report having high levels of depressive symptoms and having engaged in NSSI. Those fitting this profile also reported having lower levels of well-being at a one-year follow-up (Burke et al., 2018). Findings suggest that the dampening of positive effect can be an indicator of future NSSI. Those who engage in dampening are actively trying to reduce the intensity and duration of any positive mood experience. The reasoning behind this would be important to explore with adolescent clients. However, given that adolescents are engaged in identity development, their insight regarding the reasoning behind any positive mood dampening may be difficult to verbalize. Creative techniques can include sandtray, art, or role-play, which may assist adolescents in evaluating their reasoning while practicing self-monitoring skills.

Clinical reflection

For each client, the counselors must first assess the client's readiness for change—how willing is the individual to change the self-injurious behavior? Using the transtheoretical model is an excellent way to conceptualize readiness and apply appropriate interventions aimed at one of three goals: motivation to change, insight, and action. For those in pre-contemplation and contemplation, motivationally oriented interventions may be most useful to build a foundation for therapeutic buy-in. Once a client is contemplating change, insight-building interventions will assist clients in understanding what factors might be influencing their self-injurious behaviors. Finally, once clients begin to move into preparation for change, you can begin to transition or add in action-oriented techniques that might require practice activities outside of the counseling environment. If a client is not ready to change, it is not reasonable for a clinician to expect a client to begin practicing change in a manner that would lead to long-term behavioral improvement. This is specifically relevant to adolescent clients through adulthood, as they have more awareness and control over their life experience. The previous chapter focused more on early childhood experience and parenting, as younger children are less cognitively aware or able to communicate their intentions.

In the next section, we briefly outline one client-specific treatment goal that might be useful for each client described in this chapter (see Table 2.1). However, these goals are specifically focused on what might be the most prevalent issue intersecting with the self-injurious behavior based on the information provided. Clinicians working with clients who self-injure will likely develop three to four short-term goals based on client diagnosis and presenting concerns, and then they would re-evaluate these goals every three to six months or as needed. Additionally, clinicians may still want to include one family-oriented or parenting-oriented goal depending on the client's age, cognitive ability, and living situation. Techniques are contextualized within the transtheoretical model of change to ensure the approach is relevant to client readiness for change (e.g., meeting clients where they are).

Emma seems to have a lack of readiness for change, as evidenced by her statement that people around her need to "accept" her behaviors and not "freak out" about them. Thus, the clinician's primary task will be seeking investment for change. Motivational interviewing techniques have been demonstrated to assist clients in recognizing the potential seriousness of their self-destructive behaviors. Thus, the conversation should be focused on Emma's ambivalence toward changing her self-injurious behaviors and on behaviors she might be interested in changing. The

Table 2.1 Treatment goals

Client	*Short-term objective*	*Measure*	*Intervention*	*Readiness change*
Emma	Identify and communicate emotions linked to self-injurious behaviors.	Emotional Regulation Questionnaire (ERQ; Gross & John, 2003	1. Motivational interviewing to address investment in changing self-injurious behaviors 2. DBT strategies to understand and label emotions (e.g., STOPP)	Pre-contemplation
Rick	Increase ability to recognize his reality in terms of what he can control and what his limits are and accurately communicate with peers, teachers, and family regarding his situationally specific needs.	Interpersonal Emotional Regulation Questionnaire (IERQ; Hofmann, Carpenter, & Curtiss, 2016)	1. DBT radical acceptance 2. Cost-benefit analysis 3. Interpersonal effectiveness skills (e.g., DEAR MAN)	Contemplation
Charlotte	Self-acceptance: identify strengths and barriers to valuing aspects of her identity while valuing her emotional experience.	Cognitive Emotional Regulation Questionnaire (CERQ; Garnefski & Kraaij, 2007)	1. Narrative exposure therapy 2. DBT distress tolerance (e.g., opposite action and check the facts, wise mind ACCEPTS) 3. Acceptance-based emotional regulation group	Relapse and Preparation

discussion should link the motivation for making those changes to issues related to the self-injury (when appropriate). The goal should not be to persuade Emma why she needs to change, but to assist her in discovering her desire or reasoning for making a change. Part of the issue could be Emma's lack of emotional awareness or ability to communicate her emotional experience verbally to others. Thus, a conjoint focus on emotional understanding and labeling could assist Emma in gaining insight about a need for change and communicate that in counseling. As with any counseling process, goal achievement must be objectively and subjectively monitored. The Emotional Regulation Questionnaire (ERQ; Gross & John, 2003) is a 10-item scale that might provide some insight into how Emma experiences and expresses her emotions. This assessment will serve two functions: (1) assist Emma in thinking about and communicating her emotional process, and (2) monitor the effectiveness of emotional awareness interventions on Emma's ability to respond to items, cognitively process her emotional experience, and express those emotions (rather than suppress them).

Rick seems to recognize that he is in distress and perhaps not able to cope adequately or in the way he would like. He is relying on friends and emotionally distancing himself from his family; however, it seems he does this to avoid conflict. It may be that Rick is not able to find a method to communicate how he feels in a manner that allows him to be heard. Thus, he has difficulty expressing and regulating his emotional experience within the context of his important relationships. He works hard to suppress his feelings and uses self-injury in a way consistent with gender normative expectations (e.g., fighting and scarification) to control them. Rick may not perceive emotional communication to be beneficial to him or others. Therefore, encouraging identification and acceptance of his emotions, in conjunction with an ability to analyze the healthiest situations in which to express them, may assist Rick in communicating his feelings without resorting to self-injury. The Intrapersonal Emotional Regulation Questionnaire (IERQ; Hofmann, Carpenter, & Curtiss, 2016) consists of 20 items measuring positive affect, perspective taking, soothing, and social modeling. Normative studies included a sample population of adults consistent with demographic population statistics within the United States. As social support seems to influence Rick's emotional well-being, and self-injury tends to occur interpersonally, monitoring interpersonal emotional regulation throughout treatment may be a useful way to measure goal achievement objectively.

Charlotte has experienced successful outcomes through counseling in the past and seems to be ready to stop her self-injurious behaviors, as she had worked toward and achieved this goal in treatment previously. Given her readiness, she is likely to respond well to both insight-oriented and behaviorally oriented techniques. Charlotte indicated she has not previously processed or addressed her childhood trauma experience in counseling and seems to have issues about her self-concept. Thus, it may be helpful for Charlotte to evaluate her strengths and challenges from a narrative life history perspective to address both developmental and trauma-related perceptions of identity within a strengths-based contextual framework. Participation in an acceptance-based emotional regulation group may also assist Charlotte in building much-needed social support systems within the therapeutically guided environment so Charlotte can practice and process communicating her internal struggles with identity. As Charlotte seems to self-injure in response to perceived negative situations or events (e.g., her parents' announcement they intended to visit her at school), monitoring her cognitive coping strategies may be an effective way to objectively measure progress toward her treatment goals (see Linehan, 2017, video cited in resources). The Cognitive Emotion Regulation Questionnaire (CERQ; Garnefski et al., 2001) measures cognitive coping following negative event experience. This measure could also serve to help build Charlotte's insight related to her coping process, and thus might assist Charlotte with her self-monitoring. Additionally, using some cognitive mapping strategies could help prepare Charlotte to change some of her behavior patterns during her perceived negative events (see Appendix D).

REFERENCES

Baker, L.M., Williams, L.M., Korgaonkar, M.S., Cohen, R.A., Heaps, J.M., & Paul, R.H. (2013). Impact of early vs. late childhood early life stress on brain morphometrics. *Brain Imaging and Behavior*, 7(2), 196–203. doi:10.1007/s11682-012-9215-y

Benau, E.M., Jenkins, A.L., & Conner, B.T. (2017). Perceived parental monitoring and sexual orientation moderate lifetime acts of non-suicidal self-injury. *Archives of Suicide Research*, 21(2), 322–340. doi:10.1080/13811118.2016.1182092

Bilodeau, B.L., & Renn, K.A. (2005). Analysis of LGBT identity development models and implications for practice [PDF file]. *New Directions for Human Services*, 111. Retrieved from https://msu.edu/~renn/BilodeauRennNDSS.pdf

Brausch, A.M., & Muehlenkamp, J.J. (2018). Perceived effectiveness of NSSI in achieving functions on severity and suicide risk. *Psychiatry Research*, 265, 144–150. doi:10.1016/j.psychres.2018.04.038

Burke, T.A., Anne McArthur, B., Daryanani, I., Abramson, L.Y., & Alloy, L.B. (2018). Latent classes of trait affect and cognitive affective regulation strategies are associated with depression, non-suicidal self-injury, and well-being. *Journal of Affective Disorders*, 225, 180–187. doi:10.1016/j.jad.2017.08.015

Cervantes, R.C., Goldbach, J.T., Varela, A., & Santisteban, D.A. (2014). Self-harm among Hispanic adolescents: Investigating the role of culture-related stressors. *Journal of Adolescent Health*, 55(5), 633–639. doi:10.1016/j.jadohealth.2014.05.017

Center for Disease Control and Prevention. (2016). 10 leading causes of death by age group. National Vital Statistics System. Retrieved from https://www.cdc.gov/injury/wisqars/pdf/leading_causes_of_death_by_age_group_2016-508.pdf

Chesin, M.S., Moster, A.N., & Jeglic, E.L. (2013). Non-suicidal self-injury among ethnically and racially diverse emerging adults: Do factors unique to the minority experience matter? *Current Psychology*, 32(4), 318–328. doi:10.1007/s12144-013-9185-2

Cornell University. (2019). Self-injury and recovery research and resources (SIRRR). Retrieved from http://www.selfinjury.bctr.cornell.edu/

D'Augelli, A.R. (1994). Identity development and sexual orientation: Toward a model of lesbian, gay, and bisexual development. In: E.J. Trickett, R.J. Watts, & D. Birman (Eds.), *The Jossey-Bass Social and Behavioral Science Series. Human Diversity: Perspectives on People in Context* (pp. 312–333). San Francisco, CA: Jossey-Bass.

Garnefski, N., & Kraaij, V. (2007). The cognitive emotion regulation questionnaire. *European Journal of Psychological Assessment*, 23(3), 141–149. doi: org/10.1027/1015-5759.23.3.141

Garnefski, N., Kraaij, V., & Spinhoven, P. (2001). Negative life events, cognitive emotion regulation, and emotional problems. *Personality and Individual Differences*, 30, 1311–1327. doi:10.1016/S0191-8869(00)00113-6

Gross, J.J., & John, O.P. (2003). Individual differences in two emotion regulation processes: Implications for affect, relationships, and well-being. *Journal of Personality and Social Psychology*, 85, 348–362. doi:10.1037/0022-3514.85.2.348

Hack, J., & Graham, M. (2018). Expressed emotion, shame, and non-suicidal self-injury. *International Journal of Environmental Research and Public Health*, 15(5), 890. http://dx.doi.org.proxy.libraries.uc.edu/10.3390/ijerph15050890

Healey, A., Trepal, H., & Emelianchik-Key, K. (2010). Nonsuicidal self-injury: Examining the relationship between diagnosis and gender. *Journal of Mental Health Counseling*, 32(4), 324–341. doi:10.17744/mehc.32.4.366740506r458202

Hofmann, S.G., Carpenter, J.K., & Curtiss, J. (2016). Interpersonal Emotion Regulation Questionnaire (IERQ): Scale development and psychometric characteristics. *Cognitive Theory and Research*, 40, 341–356. doi:10.1007/s10608-016-9756-2

Kaess, M., Parzer, P., Mattern, M., Plener, P.L., Bifulco, A., Resch, F., & Brunner, R. (2013). Adverse childhood experiences and their impact on frequency, severity, and the individual function of nonsuicidal self-injury in youth. *Psychiatry Research*, 206(2–3), 265–272. doi:10.1016/j.psychres.2012.10.012

Kahn, A., McCormack, H.C., Bolger, E.A., McGreenery, C.E., Vitaliano, G., Polcari, A., & Teicher, M.H. (2015). Childhood maltreatment, depression, and suicidal ideation: Critical importance of parental and peer emotional abuse during developmental sensitive periods in males and females. *Frontiers in Psychiatry*, 6(42), 1–30. doi:10.3389/fpsyt.2015.00042

Linehan, M. [Marsha Linehan]. (2017, April 14). *How She Learned Radical Acceptance* [Video file]. Retrieved from https://youtu.be/OTG7YEWkJFI

Marchetto, M.J. 2006. Repetitive skin cutting: Parental bonding, personality and gender. *Psychology and Psychotherapy*, 79(3), 445–459. doi:10.1348/147608305X69795

Swanell, S.V., Martin, G.E., Page, A., Hasking, P. (2014). Prevalence of nonsuicidal self-injury in nonclinical samples: Systematic review, meta-analysis, and meta-regression. *Suicide and Life Threatening Behavior*, 44(3), 273–303. doi:10.1111/sltb.12070

Taliaferro, L.A., & Muehlenkamp, J.J. (2017). Nonsuicidal self-injury and suicidality among sexual minority youth: Risk factors and protective connectedness factors. *Academic Pediatrics*, 17(7), 715–722. doi:10.1016/j.acap.2016.11.002

Turner, B.J., Austin, S.B., & Chapman, A.L. (2014). Treating nonsuicidal self-injury: A systematic review of psychological and pharmacological interventions. *Can Journal Psychiatry*, 59(11), 576–585.

Victor, S.E., Hipwell, A.E., Stepp, S.D., & Scott, L.N. (2019). Parent and peer relationships as longitudinal predictors of adolescent non-suicidal self-injury onset. *Child and Adolescent Psychiatry and Mental Health*, 13(1), 1–13. doi:10.1186/s13034-018-0261-0

Zayas, L.H., Bright, C.L., Álvarez-Sánchez, T., & Cabassa, L.J. (2009). Acculturation, familism and mother-daughter relations among suicidal and non-suicidal adolescent Latinas. *Journal of Primary Prevention*, 30(3–4), 351–369. doi:10.1007/s10935-009-0181-0

3 NSSI in adulthood and aging populations

Amanda La Guardia

Youth, adults, and older adults may engage in self-injurious behaviors for differing reasons. Adults who practice self-injury (aged 30 and older) often have utilized NSSI as a child or young adult in order to manage emotions or relationships. When faced with similar distress in the future, and with little access to coping resources, these individuals may go back to self-injury to manage their distress. Adults who engage in NSSI typically do so to regulate negative affect (e.g., to release emotional pressure or to stop bad feelings) and, to a lesser extent, for self-punishment and interpersonal influence. This pattern is consistent with research that suggests that in the United States, adults in the community tend to engage in NSSI for similar reasons as adolescents (e.g., Laye-Gindhu & Schonert-Reichl, 2005; Nock & Prinstein, 2004), university students (e.g., Klonsky, 2009), and adult psychiatric patients (Briere & Gil, 1998). Gregg et al. (2018) completed a comparison study with older and younger adult veterans to assess differences in the behavior between these populations. They observed that lifetime and recent NSSI events were lower among older adult veterans. They also noted that the method of injury differed between the groups involved in the study, in that younger individuals engaged in more wall punching and cutting, while self-hitting, scratching, and burning were observed at similar rates. Thus, signs and assessments demonstrated as effective with adolescents and younger adults may be useful in determining needs for middle-aged and older adults.

Given the span of ages and developmental stages represented in the adult group, we discuss non-suicidal self-injury related to three cases to provide a variety of examples, thus highlighting the expansive needs of this group. Each of these cases will be conceptualized using current research indicators for risk and protective factors (which will be reviewed in more depth in Part II) while integrating evidence-based and professionally accepted practices. When attempting to cope with emergent life stressors, adults have a lifetime of experiences to draw upon; however, some of those skills may not be healthy, and the willingness to change behavioral patterns is sometimes low due to the desire to maintain equilibrium or to stick to what one knows. The design of our brains allows us to build upon and protect habits that make us feel good, which sometimes gets in the way of meaningful change (see Ryback, 2017, "Neurobiology of Change"). Thus, promoting and maintaining change can be difficult, especially when the change involves an entrenched, long-standing habit that works, like non-suicidal self-injury.

Case 3.1: Case of Jimmy

Jimmy is a 55-year-old Black, straight male struggling with recent alcohol abuse who has a history of narcotics abuse and untreated intermittent NSSI throughout his life. He has never sought support or help for substance abuse. He reports struggling with suicidal ideation off and on, but he has not attempted suicide since his early 20s. He has been married for 15 years and has no children. His relationship with his spouse is great (as reported by Jimmy) when he is not drinking. He reports that his spouse is supportive and says she urged him to seek help for what is "bothering him" because she thinks it is "hurting" their relationship. He is not sure how a counselor can help and does not believe in mental health care as important for health but does come in to see you to please his wife. He believes he should be able to handle his issues. He also asserts that relational problems should be handled in the family. Jimmy says to you, "I am fine, and I have been managing as best I can over the years." It is evident that he is not in denial of the present issues, but he believes that he is "fine" since there has not been recent suicidal ideation or attempts. Jimmy reports he self-injured after an argument with his spouse a few weeks ago. He was drunk. He said he got very angry because he was worried his wife was going to leave him. After the argument, he laid his hand on the stovetop for a couple of seconds, knowing it was still hot from cooking a recent meal. He said the burn helped him to calm down and that "it is better I do that than yell more at my wife or break something." He did not think the injury was very severe and did not seek medical attention. He said this incident is what prompted his spouse to push for counseling. Jimmy initially agrees to meet with you for four sessions every other week and will then decide on the continuation of services. He is very ambivalent about making any changes in his behavior, but he recognizes there are things that "could be better."

Developmental perspective

While adults are cognitively able to process information in logical and abstract ways, concrete thinking can occur in times of stress or due to trauma-related stress. Trauma can *derail* processing and result in apprehension toward problem-solving, attachment problems, or distress around authority figures or particular environments. These psychosocial consequences can persist long into adulthood. Substance use can also influence cognitive processing. As Jimmy is in his mid-50s, he is capable of thinking creatively, can empathize with others, and strategize about the future. However, he may have emotional difficulties and internalized beliefs about himself and others that make these ways of thinking more difficult. Jimmy falls within the generativity versus the stagnation stage, where he needs to feel like he has contributed to society and the world in some way and to derive a sense of purpose through family, work, or other means. Psychosocially, Jimmy is in a stage of his life when the mid-life crisis is common. He may be attempting to find a sense of purpose within his family, and he needs to generate a sense of societal and/or relational worth to experience a broader meaning for living. Exploring how Jimmy finds purpose and meaning in his life is a developmentally appropriate way to address issues that may be contributing to his self-injurious behaviors and alcohol abuse.

Diversity issues

A number of cultural factors could influence Jimmy's reticence to seek mental health treatment. Jimmy stated some values that provide some clues as to his perspective on his cultural experiences, namely his belief that individuals should be able to handle their issues and that problems in the family should be discussed and resolved within the family. When thinking about cultural stigma related to mental health care, Yang et al. (2014) propose a "what matters most" perspective, suggesting that "culture affects stigma by threatening an actor's capacity to participate in the activities that determine 'what matters most' (or 'personhood') within a cultural context" (p. 496). In Jimmy's case, he may perceive help-seeking for his internal struggles as a threat to his ability to take care of himself, or his mental strength, which may pose a threat to what he expects of himself as a man within his cultural context. Hence, he may believe that help-seeking about problems within his intimate relationship speaks to his ability to be a leader within his home. One typically accesses mental health care institutionally (through community agencies or hospitals), and the profession itself is regulated. Thus, Jimmy could perceive seeking care as a potential threat to his independence due to historical and present-day issues regarding institutionalized oppression. All of these factors possibly influence his decision to engage in "four sessions" before fully committing to the process. The fact that Jimmy is in counseling at all speaks to his readiness and willingness to challenge himself—as well as culturally influenced beliefs—in order to make a change. Apprehension about mental health care should not be conflated with apprehension toward engaging actively in change.

Risk and protective factors

Jimmy revealed that he struggled with narcotics abuse and alcohol abuse early in his life, which may be reflective of early adulthood distress. In a 15-year longitudinal study of men, those who identified as Black and engaged in early-life heavy drinking were thought to have experienced higher levels of distress associated with the heavy drinking. These individuals were more likely to experience deleterious mid-life outcomes, particularly with regard to employment and perceived occupational success (Sloan et al., 2011). It may be useful to explore some of Jimmy's early life stressors and his occupational satisfaction, given his developmental stage and current coping with relational distress. While the self-injury seems impulsive and purposeful, the alcohol abuse may be a habitual way of coping that is based on a belief that life will be distressing; thus, this method assists him in avoiding the full experience of his distress (preventative emotional regulation). NSSI and substance abuse have been linked in some research studies, and this finding tends to indicate that increased distress and risk for suicide, as well as unintentional severe injury when self-injuring, occur concurrently with substance use. Given Jimmy's history of suicidal ideation and suicidal attempts, his risk for suicide is even greater. Therefore, the combination of these behaviors is of great concern, and issues contributing to these coping methods should be the primary focus of treatment.

Jimmy's focus on self-reliance is a personal and cultural strength that will benefit engagement in treatment and assist in motivating lasting change. Encouraging social support through culturally non-threatening avenues (e.g., religious communities, supportive and healthy family relationships, or trusted community groups) may allow Jimmy to seek external assistance when needed, but in a way that does not threaten his self-reliance. Healing can occur through engagement in healthy supportive relationships, whether that happens in the counseling room or outside of it. Jimmy seems to perceive his intimate partnership as healthy, and his wife's urging for him to seek help indicates that she is invested in his growth. Her support and his connection to her may serve to assist Jimmy as he works toward making and maintaining change. Engaging her in session as a support could be a useful component of any goal, consistent with Jimmy's desire to solve relational problems within the family. By interpreting her involvement as a way of maintaining any gains made in counseling within the home, Jimmy may become more motivated to make supportive changes (e.g., reducing alcohol consumption and engaging in healthy communication). Ultimately, if he is appropriately able to express many of his internal struggles to his partner rather than suppressing them, some of the relational distress he is experiencing may resolve.

Case 3.2: Case of Rhonda

Rhonda is a White, 35-year-old, recently divorced female with a history of domestic violence victimization. Rhonda married at 18 and had her first child by the age of 19. After caring for her three children over the past 15 years, she is currently re-entering the workforce outside of the home. She is confident in her decision to leave her abusive relationship, but she is scared since she now must financially support herself and her children. Rhonda reports a history of adolescent self-injury, which she says she stopped engaging in when she was in her early to mid-20s. Rhonda is very worried that her children might be negatively affected by her absence due to employment and is concerned about her ability to retain a job. She has been employed in her current position for six months but lost her previous job "because of problems with anxiety" that resulted in her leaving work or calling in sick frequently. Rhonda has been thinking about self-injuring again and has been "trying not to do it," engaging in the behavior "infrequently" and only with "little cuts" as the pain from the cutting helps her to "calm down." Rhonda is particularly concerned about how her absence from the home will affect her youngest child, who is eight. She says her oldest, aged 15, is not trustworthy and has frequent anger outbursts. She is concerned about the time her children will be alone between the end of the school day and her arrival home from work in the evening. Rhonda states that she is also highly anxious that the children's father will find them and kidnap her children or harm them while she is at work. Rhonda says her anxiety is extremely distracting and when it overwhelms her, the only way she knows to deal with it is by cutting. Rhonda comes to counseling on Saturdays and leaves her children in the waiting room during sessions with an adult friend. Rhonda is seeing a psychiatrist and has been prescribed Wellbutrin. She reports that the medication she receives seems to help her to feel better in general but does not help her when she has "a wave of worry." Rhonda believes her anxiety is justified, due to her circumstances, and wants to stop her self-injury, as she fears her oldest will begin to notice and engage in the behavior as well. Ultimately, Rhonda would like to manage her anxiety better, but her current focus is on reducing her self-injury.

Developmental perspective

Individuals in their 30s face psychosocial challenges within the stage of intimacy versus isolation. This phase is marked by a process of attempting to find balance in one's sense of self through relationships and finding a sense of self through introspection. During this time, an individual establishes personal boundaries, evaluates those boundaries, and sometimes changes them to ensure relationships are personally meaningful and that one feels understood and accepted by others. Thus, the relational self can be a primary focus in the process of identity growth. For more information about factors that characterize the relational self, see Chen et al. (2011). Rhonda began the intimacy versus isolation stage of development by getting married at age 18. She likely did not have a strong grasp over her identity within her previous stage of development, which allowed her to question herself and stay with someone dominant and abusive. Without a strong sense of identity, it was hard for Rhonda to build the courage to stand up to her abusive partner. Tolerance of abuse in intimate relationships is also viewed as a form of indirect self-harm, as the person allows it to continue and feels like it is deserved. When Rhonda was finally able to leave her abusive partner, she was able to overcome the potential fear that comes along with isolation. Ultimately, Rhonda will need to explore her self-regulatory strategies and behavioral motivations and make connections to the way they are influenced by her self-concept and ways of relating to others in significant relationships.

Diversity issues

In thinking about self-injury, it may be helpful to attend to potential gender differences in the presentation of the behavior. Bresin and Schoenleber (2015) evaluated the prevalence of NSSI methods across 122 studies. Women engaged in significantly more cutting, biting, scratching, hair pulling, and wound interference (methods that generally involve blood). Men were slightly more inclined to engage in burning, hitting, and banging. In this analysis, women were 1.5 times more likely than men to report NSSI behaviors, but this overall difference was small, with no significant differences between men and women in community and college samples included in the meta-analysis. Addressing why an individual seeks treatment may help clinicians to understand the reason for the self-injury better. Understanding differences in presentation of NSSI methods allows us to recognize how different cultural messages about gender normative behaviors may translate to symptomology (i.e., cutting versus hitting).

Rhonda appears to identify with the dominant ethnic culture; however, values specific to her family may indicate that cultural influences are not readily stated. Often, White individuals will struggle to identify a culture of influence, but these may exist within faith communities, regional upbringing, and persistent generational and cultural traditions. Due to societal privilege, White individuals may have little to no motivation to explore their values in a way that leads to specific cultural identification, as this is not necessary to create or preserve an appreciation of self through a sense of culturally specific collective safety or belongingness. White individuals experience safety and development of self through acceptance from dominant cultural norms and privileges. However, exploration of beliefs and values may facilitate insight, contributing to a foundation for the development of healthy coping skills. This could begin with a discussion of how cultural norms influence perceptions of self. In Rhonda's case, this could include her perceptions of what it means to be a mother, as this role seems to contribute to her current anxiety (e.g., her need to protect her children from their abusive father). Rhonda may also need to explore what it means to be female and a "wife" or her role as a female in an intimate relationship. Inherited gender messages that could be generational might contribute to her staying in an abusive relationship for so long. Additionally, her decision to stay could have been mediated through her desire to regulate her emotions through indirect means of self-injury. Through an exploration of her values, beliefs, and gender messages, we can identify cognitive distortions that might be present and developmental challenges that could be holding Rhonda back in successfully overcoming her NSSI. Additionally, this will allow Rhonda to identify strengths she could use to motivate and support her desired change and move forward.

Risk and protective factors

Rhonda cares deeply for her children and is motivated to change her self-injurious behavior; however, she seems to feel somewhat hopeless concerning her anxiety. She appears to be living in a state of fear, which may be triggering survival-based anxieties similar to what she likely experienced during intimate partner abuse. Smith et al. (2014) completed a systematic review of NSSI and trauma literature, showing a potential conceptual mediating role of trauma symptomology in the relationship between traumatic experiences and self-injury. In Rhonda's case, the proposed model helps to explain the resurgence of her self-injurious behavior. Further, the model, if accurate, would seem to suggest that treatment of her trauma symptoms might be important in ultimately stopping her self-injurious behaviors. However, this issue is complex, as Rhonda seems to find value in her anxiety at present and is reticent to address it. Nevertheless, she is motivated to stop her self-injury, so it may be prudent to start using motivational interviewing techniques with a goal she is ready to address, as a way to examine the deeper issue and ensure the successful cessation of the self-injury. Rhonda appears to have at least one close friend and is financially stable. Exploring her tangible and intangible resources would be beneficial to help Rhonda evaluate her support system and develop a stronger sense of safety around her ability to protect herself and her family.

TEXTBOX 3.1 REFLECTING ON TRAUMA EXPERIENCE AND NSSI

In a study by Silva et al. (2017), a model was analyzed and indicated that emotional regulation difficulties fully mediated the relationship between non-suicidal self-injury and dimensions of current or past unhealthy romantic relationships (including intimate partner violence, abandonment anxiety, and avoidance of intimacy). This means that while traumatic relational events may influence the onset of NSSI, the emotional dysregulation of the individual explains maintenance of self-injurious behaviors.

Given this information, how might you prioritize treatment of non-suicidal self-injury in cases involving a traumatic event or trauma history as a precursor to NSSI behaviors?

Source: Silva, E., Machado, B.C., Moreira, C.S., Ramalho, S., & Gonçalves, S. (2017). Romantic relationships and nonsuicidal self-injury among college students: The mediating role of emotion regulation. *Journal of Applied Developmental Psychology*, 50, 36–44. doi:10.1016/j.appdev.2017.04.001

Case 3.3: Case of Dean

Dean is a 68-year-old, White male whose partner recently passed from colon cancer. He has a history of non-suicidal self-injury and alcohol abuse dating back to adolescence. Currently, he is struggling to cope with the loss of his partner of 20 years. He was diagnosed with Parkinson's disease five years ago and is concerned about his ability to care for himself in the future. His partner was a constant source of support and the "only one that knew" about his lifetime struggles with NSSI. He identifies as Episcopalian and states his faith is very important to him. Dean reports his church community was previously a "central part" of his life when his partner was alive; however, Dean has had difficulty going to church since his death. He does not know "where to start with all of the health difficulties" in his own life, and he does not feel like going to church or engaging with other people will be helpful to him. He feels like a burden to his old friends and does not want to have to "put all of" his "problems on them." Dean reports to be actively self-injuring and has visible bruising and scars on his arms. He says he will hit his arms against the wall or any hard object nearby when he starts to "feel like" he is "losing control" of his movements. He believes this helps him to stay calm but also helps him to "regain control for a moment." Dean was referred to counseling by his neurologist. He currently takes the medication Cogentin and vitamin E supplements. Dean reports that he is not taking any medication for depression and has not done so "for a number of years." He reports that his doctor attempted to prescribe medication to help with the depressive symptoms, but Dean refused because he believes his "depression is normal given all of the problems I'm having" and does not want "some drug messing with" his brain. He fears adding more medication will somehow worsen the progression of his Parkinson's. He is willing to work in counseling to address his feelings of sadness, isolation, and anxiety about his future.

Developmental perspective

Individuals aged 60 and older are considered to be in the psychosocial phase of integrity versus despair, which means that Dean is likely in a period of reflection upon his life and evaluating his accomplishments concerning his expectations. He may feel a sense of regret about the past, unfulfilled in some way related to his life thus far, and a sense of loss regarding plans and expectations he had for the future. The loss of his primary support system and partner of 20 years may be exacerbating a sense of despair about the end of his life. Additionally, his Parkinson's symptoms further complicate his grief, as he loses physical function and potentially his independence. While Dean's stage of Parkinson's is unclear, it is likely he is early in the development of symptoms (stage one or two). At an early stage, it is unlikely the progression of the disease is influencing cognitive functioning or psychological symptomology directly. The primary developmental concern seems to be related to end-of-life meaning-making and future planning in relation to the prognosis of Dean's Parkinson's diagnosis.

Diversity issues

Dean identifies as a gay man. He also identifies as Episcopalian and was active in his faith community prior to his partner's death. As a gay male, Dean is likely to experience higher levels of minority stress and gender role conflict in relation to his NSSI behaviors. Males are less likely to seek out mental health services due to the stigma that surrounds societal constructs of what it means to be a "man." Dean has struggled with lifetime NSSI. We are not sure if he has engaged in any treatment, nor do we know the ways that gender role conflict affects Dean. If he is a traditional male, he could be very proud, and events that come along with aging, like retirement, loss of purpose, loss of cognition, and other physical and mental impairments, could be significantly impacting his cognitions and emotionality.

Additionally, non-dominant sexual groups are at an increased risk for NSSI and often more frequent and severe NSSI behaviors because of minority stress (Fox et al., 2018). Shame is also an indirect factor associated with NSSI. We do not know if Dean is an openly gay male, but if he is experiencing shame or has in the past, this could be contributing to his NSSI behaviors. We do know that being a self-injurer has caused Dean shame, as his partner was the only person who knew he self-injured. Additionally, discrimination, oppression, bullying, social isolation, microaggression, and prejudice all contribute to NSSI. We are not aware of how he has handled being a gay male, nor if he is out to his community and his church community. The Episcopalian faith is known for accepting all sexual orientations as "God's children" since 1976. However, with Dean being 68 years old, this acceptance has likely not been experienced his whole life. It is highly probable that Dean has faced discrimination and oppression from many people in the past, including people of his faith, which could all affect his NSSI behaviors. Dean may once again be challenged by parts of his faith and spiritual identity as he faces a progressive health disorder, which is not terminal but could cause excruciating pain and loss of functionality. If he does get to the point of facing end-of-life decisions, his faith could add to his distress and conflict in making end-of-life decisions. Dean will need to work with a counselor who has competence and understanding of faith-based practices so they can help him integrate and be at peace with future decisions regarding his illness.

Risk and protective factors

Older adults have higher rates of death by suicide than any other age group, with those who are 45 to 54 having the highest rates, followed by 85 and older, 55 to 64, and 75 to 84 (AFSP, 2019). While Dean is not in those age ranges, his health prognosis and mental health history heighten his risk for suicide. Assessment of his support system, as it stands, will be critical to understanding Dean's therapeutic needs. Dean seems reluctant to engage with his prior friend group due to fears of becoming a burden. Thus, it is likely effective to broach the topic of social reengagement from a grief-based and motivational perspective, honoring Dean's beliefs and experiences. Gradual exploration and *testing of the waters* may assist Dean in opening up to one or two of his closest friends.

Religiosity has been shown to serve as a protective factor for suicide, perhaps due to the sense of connectedness and belongingness that can come with strong ties to a faith community. Values related to life and suicide may play a role in preventing suicidal behavior through social pressures to conform to doctrine. However, the process by which religion serves as a protective factor is unclear. According to Joiner's (2009) Interpersonal Theory of Suicide, a lack of belongingness, sense of burdensomeness, and ability to act intersect to create heightened suicide risk severity. Dean's re-engagement with his faith community may help to prevent escalation of symptom experience related to his growing sense of isolation and anxiety about the future.

Conclusion

Non-suicidal self-injury is a serious concern for older adults that is overlooked in the NSSI literature. In a study by Choi et al. (2016) of older adults admitted to emergency departments, NSSI was found to be highly associated with higher hospitalization and death rates than suicide attempts. The researchers cautioned that intentional self-destructive behaviors later in life could be of great concern and potentially lethal, even if not classified as a suicide attempt. They included approximately 67,000 people in their study and found NSSI rates of 23% within this sample population. These results serve to highlight how clinically relevant and important this problem is for older individuals struggling with developmental challenges and mental health issues that may trigger the onset and maintenance of NSSI. For more information on the needs of older adults in relation to suicidal behaviors, please see Deuter and Procter (2015).

Clinical reflections

Similar to clinical work with adolescents and young adults, an adult or older adult has to have buy-in for change. However, in later adulthood, individuals may have developed more entrenched patterns and reasoning associated with the justification of their self-injury. Thus, assessment for change readiness is still essential to appropriate intervention decisions designed to address NSSI behaviors directly or indirectly. In developing treatment and outcomes assessment, considerations of readiness are essential (see Table 3.1).

Jimmy seems to be reluctant to engage in treatment, but he also appears to recognize that he has an issue he would like to change—namely, his impulsive self-injury and alcohol abuse. Due to contextual and cultural factors, Jimmy may appear to be contemplating change when, in fact, he may be making plans to take action for change. Thus, as a process of therapeutic engagement, Jimmy may be straddling the contemplation and preparation stages of change. Motivational interviewing techniques, like cost-benefit analysis, may be a client-centered and direct way to engage Jimmy in a treatment process slowly. Additionally, drawing upon his relationship with his wife may also assist Jimmy in feeling more comfortable with treatment while focusing on improving healthy communication of needs within his relationship, with the goal of preventing future self-injury. The AUDIT, or Alcohol Use Disorders Identification Test, is a 10-item screener used by the World Health Organization (WHO) to assess for hazardous or harmful alcohol use and has been validated with a wide range of racial and ethnic populations. This inventory may help to facilitate insight into the problem while monitoring use throughout treatment. Additionally, the SASSI-4 (Substance Abuse Subtle Screening Inventory) is an accurate measure used to predict substance use

Table 3.1 Treatment goals

Client	*Short-term objective*	*Measure*	*Intervention*	*Readiness change*
Jimmy	Evaluate the pros and cons of alcohol use and sobriety while building healthy social support in the home.	AUDIT SASSI-4	1. Cost-benefit analysis 2. DEARMAN interpersonal effectiveness training and couples work	Contemplation/ preparation
Rhonda	Reduce engagement in and urge to self-injure.	BAI CSQ-8	1. T-SIB, treatment for self-injurious behaviors 2. TIPP for anxiety management	Preparation
Dean	Reduce feelings of isolation and increase supportive network.	BDI Quality of Life Scale (QOLS)	1. Complicated Grief Treatment (CGT)	Preparation/ action

disorders, and it includes measures of defensiveness toward treatment, family systems assessment, and problem acknowledgment, among other indicators. This measure would help assess and evaluate characteristics associated with Jimmy's alcohol abuse and would be most useful if given at 6–12-month intervals to evaluate changes in his perspectives toward his alcohol abuse.

As Rhonda's primary focus is on behavioral change, she is likely in the preparation stages an individual engages in before taking action toward change. Focusing on anxiety symptom management using TIPP (Temperature, Intense Exercise, Paced Breathing, Paired Muscle Relaxation) and behavioral intervention may assist in both reducing the urge to initiate and engage in self-injury. While in-the-moment anxiety management is an important step in NSSI prevention, additional approaches are necessary to redirect feelings of anxiety and resultant self-injurious behaviors. T-SIB (Treatment for Self-Injurious Behavior) is a nine-week, one-hour session per week intervention developed by Andover et al. (2015) to address self-injurious behaviors in young adults. Given the adults in the test, the group was experiencing similar psychosocial developmental challenges; this treatment may be effective for Rhonda. The BAI (Beck Anxiety Inventory) and the CSQ-8 (client satisfaction questionnaire) may help to monitor Rhonda's anxiety and her continued interest in treatment. Providing some simple relaxation exercises for Rhonda to do when she recognizes her anxiety will assist her as she starts to develop concrete coping skills (see Appendix E for an example activity).

Dean, while seemingly ready to take action, seems to be struggling with multiple areas of grief that could be impeding his ability to plan for and invest in behavioral change. Complicated Grief Treatment has demonstrated effectiveness with individuals diagnosed with chronic, potentially terminal illnesses and addresses multiple facets of related behavioral issues (see Center for Complicated Grief, Columbia School of Social Work, 2017). The BDI (Beck Depression Inventory) and Quality of Life Scale (QOLS; Burckhardt & Anderson, 2003) may assist in assessing aspects of depression and grief associated with Dean's current isolation, loss of support network, and terminal diagnosis. Differentiating aspects of grief from depression is critical when working with terminally ill clients, as some feelings associated with Dean's diagnosis may be normal and ultimately adaptive, while others may hinder the quality of life (Widera & Block, 2012).

REFERENCES

American Foundation for Suicide Prevention. (2019). *Suicide statistics*. Retrieved from https://afsp.org/about-suicide/suicide-statistics/

Andover, M.S., Schatten, H.T., Morris, B.W., & Miller, I.W. (2015). Development of an intervention for nonsuicidal self-injury in young adults: An open pilot trial. *Cognitive and Behavioral Practice*, 22(4), 491–503. https://www.doi.org/10.1016/j.cbpra.2014.05.003

Briere, J., & Gil, E. (1998). Self-mutilation in clinical and general population samples: Prevalence, correlates, and functions. *American Journal of Othropsychiatry*, 68(4), 609–620. doi:10.1037/h0080369

Bresin, K., & Schoenleber, M. (2015). Gender differences in the prevalence of nonsuicidal self-injury: A meta-analysis. *Clinical Psychology Review*, 38, 55–64. doi:10.1016/j.cpr.2015.02.009

Burckhardt, C.S., & Anderson, K.L. (2003). The Quality of Life Scale (QOLS): Reliability, validity, and utilization. *Health and Quality of Life Outcomes*, 1, 60. doi:10.1186/1477–7525-1-60

Chen S., Boucher H., & Kraus M.W. (2011). The relational self. In: S. Schwartz, K. Luyckx, & V. Vignoles. *Handbook of Identity Theory and Research* (pp. 149–175). New York, NY: Springer.

Choi, B.Y., Choi, N.G., DiNitto, D.M., & Marti, C.N. (2016). Nonsuicidal self-injury and suicide attempts among ED patients older than 50 years: Comparison of risk factors and ED visit outcomes. *American Journal of Emergency Medicine*, 34(6), 1016–1021. doi:10.1016/j.ajem.2016.02.058

Columbia School of Social Work. (2017). The Center for Complicated Grief. Retrieved from https://complicatedgrief.columbia.edu/professionals/complicated-grief-professionals/treatment/

Deuter, K., & Procter, N. (2015). Attempted suicide in older people: A review of the evidence. *Suicidologi*, 20(3). doi:10.5617/suicidologi.2636

Fox, K.R., Hooley, J.M., Smith, D.M., Ribeiro, J.D., Huang, X., Nock, M.K., & Franklin, J.C. (2018). Self-injurious thoughts and behaviors may be more common and severe among people identifying as a sexual minority. *Behavior Therapy*, 49(5), 768–780. doi:10.1016/j.beth.2017.11.009

Gregg, J., Deming, C., Libman, C., Clancy, C., Calhoun, P., Beckham, J., & Kimbrel, N. (2018). Nonsuicidal self-injury in older versus middle-aged/younger veterans seeking treatment for posttraumatic stress. *Innovation in Aging*, 2(1), 972. doi:10.1093/geroni/igy031.3600

Joiner, T. (2009). The interpersonal-psychological theory of suicidal behavior: Current empirical status. *Psychological Science Agenda: Science Briefs*. Retrieved from https://www.apa.org/science/about/psa/2009/06/sci-brief

Klonsky, E.D. (2009). The functions of self-injury in young adults who cut themselves: Clarifying the evidence for affect-regulation. *Psychiatry Research*, 166(2–3), 260–268. doi:10.1016/j.psychres.2008.02.008

Laye-Gindhu, A., & Schonert-Reichl, K.A. (2005). Nonsuicidal self-harm among community adolescents: Understanding the "whats" and "whys" of self-harm. *Journal of Youth Adolescence*, 34(5), 447–457. doi:10.1007/s10964.005.7262.z

Nock, M.K., & Prinstein, M.J. (2004). A functional approach to the assessment of self-mutilative behavior. *Journal of Consulting and Clinical Psychology*, 72(5), 885–890. doi:10.1037/0022-006X.72.5.885

Ryback, R. (2017). Why we resist change. *Psychology Today*. Retrieved from https://www.psychologytoday.com/us/blog/the-truisms-wellness/201701/why-we-resist-change

Sloan, F.A., Costanzo, P.R., Belsky, D., Holmberg, E., Malone, P.S., Wang, Y., & Kertesz, S. (2011). Heavy drinking in early adulthood and outcomes at mid life. *Journal of Epidemiology and Community Health*, 65(7), 600–605. doi:10.1136/jech.2009.102228

Smith, N.B., Kouros, C.D., & Meuret, A.E. (2014). The role of trauma symptoms in nonsuicidal self-injury. *Trauma, Violence, & Abuse*, 15(1), 41–56. doi:10.1177/1524838013496332

Widera, E.W., & Block, S.D. (2012). Managing grief and depression at the end of life. *American Family Physician*, 86(3):259–264.

Yang, L.H., Thornicroft, G., Alvarado, R., Vega, E., & Link, B.G. (2014). Recent advances in cross-cultural measurement in psychiatric epidemiology: Utilizing "what matters most" to identify culture-specific aspects of stigma. *International Journal of Epidemiology*, 43(2), 494–510. doi:10.1093/ije/dyu039

Part II

Assessment and screening for non-suicidal self-injury

Chapters in Part II review the various contexts in which NSSI occurs and clinical perspectives related to the purpose of NSSI in children, adolescents, and adults. We present conceptualizations of NSSI across the lifespan in detail, along with DSM 5 diagnostic considerations associated with the behavior. We integrate issues related to culture, identity development, gender, and function of NSSI throughout these chapters specific to assessment, interpretation, and clinical determinations for treatment. Review of formal and informal assessment techniques in addition to ways to adapt assessments per the needs of the client are applied to select cases presented in section one of the book. Case scenarios presented in Part I are used throughout Part II to highlight theoretical and procedural recommendations, while examining additional factors and information that would result from assessing and conceptualizing the client from different frameworks. We guide the reader to reflect on their own process in making appropriate clinical decisions when practicing with our unique case scenarios.

4 Risk and protective factors

Kelly Emelianchik-Key

Understanding risk and protective factors in childhood is critical for non-suicidal self-injury conceptualization, assessment, prevention, and intervention. It is useful for clinicians to think from a psychosocial and developmental framework to utilize appropriately risk and protective factor research knowledge in the treatment of NSSI and suicide-related behaviors. Neurobiological and neuropsychological perspectives add components necessary for the development of realistic, achievable, evidence-based goals and outcome monitoring. The relationship between protective factors and risk factors associated with NSSI in adolescents and young adults is difficult to predict due to the complex interactions of biological, social, and physiological complexities. Adolescence is sometimes a tumultuous time where developmental needs and changes can present a poor fit with the environment, which leads to differential experiencing of risk and protective factors. Some of the risk factors for adolescents and young adults overlap with those found in older adults, but not consistently, which highlights the need for developmentally based approaches to assess these factors. NSSI can co-occur with substance abuse, hair pulling, and eating disordered behaviors, so treatment should include the potential for other self-harming coping strategies. Throughout this section, we mention each of the risk and protective factors found in related case scenarios from earlier in the text and address how and why this information is important. We will cover practical ways to use and identify the information so that you can discern a process for identifying risk and protective factors and utilize them in client treatment.

Terminology for examining risk

The risk factors for NSSI are important to examine as they assist clinicians with developing primary, secondary, and tertiary treatments. Knowing risk factors helps clinicians when performing a risk assessment by improving a practitioner's ability to attend to potentially useful contextual information to elucidate factors important to care. To begin, it is necessary to discuss the definition of some key terms associated with this topic—risk, risk factor, correlative factor, and causal risk factor—and distinguish between them. Research literature tends to include these terms in a way that seems interchangeable, but they are not the same. *Risk* is the probability that something will happen. Defining the relationship between a factor and developing NSSI behaviors is probabilistic, not deterministic, so *risk factors* are those aspects that are measurable, precede the outcome, and make someone more likely to be associated with the higher *risk* group for developing the outcome (Kraemer et al., 1997). *Correlative factors* are the variables that have an association with the outcome, but the nature of the correlation can be vague. Kraemer et al. (1997) state that to determine a variable as a *risk factor*, it must be assessed before the outcome occurs because even though it may be a risk factor, it might be associated with the consequence (i.e., NSSI). With this in mind, the *risk* is the probability of an outcome; the *correlate* is a measure associated with the outcome; the *risk factor* is the correlate shown to precede the outcome; and the *causal risk factor* is a risk factor that, when changed, can alter the outcome (Kraemer et al., 1997). A risk factor can be changed or modified. A *predictive factor* is a likelihood that a risk factor will lead to the outcome (NSSI). Predictive factors are similar to risk factors, but they anticipate that an outcome will occur. Conversely, *protective factors* are personal or social characteristics and resources that can help a person to overcome risk factors, while also supporting a person's ability to be resilient to challenges in life (Snyder & Lopez, 2001). The reason risk factors are not predictive is because protective factors are inherent to every individual client; thus, both must be considered to determine accurate odds of a particular outcome. By helping clients identify protective factors associated with the self and other experiences, you will assist in reducing, and ultimately stopping, NSSI behaviors. At the end of this chapter, you will see a chart that maps out the risk factors and protective factors that are present in all case studies.

Risk factors

There are many risk factors associated with NSSI that overlap among children, adolescent, and adult populations engaging in self-injury. Some of the predictors and risk factors associated with NSSI onset and progression include having a history of childhood abuse and neglect, genetic factors, lack of emotional regulation strategies, parental support and communication, exposure to peer NSSI, trauma, bullying, presence of mental health conditions, and stressful life events (Arbuthnott & Lewis, 2015; Nock, 2010). The parent-child relationship has also been found to be predictive of the onset and progression of NSSI. Exposure to childhood adversity and proximal environmental adversities, such as peer groups or family difficulties, increases the risk of NSSI and mental illness (Dunn et al., 2011; van Harmelen et al., 2016). Understanding each of the individual factors that contribute to NSSI in children and adults is critical to mitigating future NSSI behaviors and suicide risk. Additionally, understanding protective factors, which will help prevent or stop a person from engaging in NSSI, is equally important.

Interpersonal and intrapersonal factors

When examining risk factors, distinguishing between intrapersonal (e.g., coping styles, emotional regulation, self-esteem, psychopathology, and depressive symptoms) and interpersonal (e.g., family abuse, parenting and attachment, and social factors) risk factors is important. Intrapersonal risk factors and NSSI are more often highlighted throughout the NSSI literature (Baetens et al., 2014), whereas interpersonal factors are examined less frequently. Intrapersonal risk factors are those aspects that a client can work toward changing. Interpersonal factors are often those elements that a client has very little to no control over changing. Beginning as early as childhood, NSSI can be utilized as a way to cope with high levels of psychological distress (Nock, 2010), which includes internalizing and externalizing symptoms (Baetens et al., 2012). Inter- and intrapersonal factors are both found to play a role in the development and maintenance of NSSI as well as potential risk for suicide.

Attachment styles and parental abuse

A practitioner may begin investigating risk factors and correlates that occurred in infancy, which is the first point in development that may be examined, as early risk factors could play a role in self-harming behaviors, including self-injury. According to Bowlby (1973), attachment theory is the relationship between the infant and caregiver, and this relationship will provide a framework for all future relationships and behaviors throughout development. Infants that are securely attached will feel worthy of support and love. They usually have a better self-concept and cope in healthier ways as they grow. Secure attachment with caregivers can serve as a protective factor for NSSI. Those infants that are insecurely attached to caregivers are more prone or susceptible to poor coping skills and poor psychological functioning later in life. These poor coping skills include self-injurious behaviors (Yates et al., 2008). It also becomes harder for these individuals to form bonds and attachments later in life. Studies have found insecure attachment styles to be most prevalent for those that engage in NSSI (Kokaliari, 2014). A poor attachment style has the potential to lead to anxiety in the parent-child relationship when children reach adolescence (West et al., 1998). Disorganized (unresolved) attachment styles are those that fall between secure and insecure attachment and are sometimes referred to as an ambivalent attachment. Parents or caregivers will meet the child's needs at times, but at other times, they act inconsistently, typically in moments of relational stress. In these moments, a child can start to fear their parent or caregiver. This leaves the child with uncertainty, and he or she may become unsure as to whether they can turn to their parent or caregiver when needed. The anxiety within the caregiver relationships (Baetens et al., 2014), and suppression and withdrawal of emotion that surrounds the relationship, opposed to effective emotion regulation, expressively increases the likelihood of NSSI engagement (Andrews et al., 2013).

Additionally, parental disapproval, criticism, abuse, and neglect in childhood and adolescence are contributing factors for NSSI onset (You & Leung, 2012). Girls who are exposed to expressions of maternal emotional criticism in childhood (ages 7–11) are more likely to engage in lifetime NSSI, as compared to boys within the same age group (James & Gibb, 2019). This suggests that either boys have some innate protective factor or girls are more sensitive to maternal critique during this period. Yates et al. (2008) also established that adults who engaged in more recurrent and extreme NSSI behaviors were those with childhood experiences of abuse/neglect from parental figures. These findings further support the notion that childhood maltreatment and abuse are strong risk factors associated with NSSI (Serafini et al., 2017). Having more consistent parental or caregiver support can help moderate the lifetime effects of abuse, maltreatment, and criticism; thus, such support may be a protective factor.

Parenting styles

There are four parenting styles: indulgent (low control with high support), authoritarian (high control with low support), authoritative (high control with high support), and uninvolved (low control and low support). Wedig and Nock (2007) found that parental criticism and hostility is a strong correlate to NSSI, while Polk and Liss (2007) noted that lack of emotional nurturance and an authoritarian parenting style are predictive of NSSI. This shows that too much of these various parenting factors predicts NSSI. Hay and Meldrum (2010) examined bullying and NSSI to find that having an authoritative parent and higher levels of self-control decreased and even eliminated the risk of NSSI engagement for those victimized through bullying. This suggests that a consistent, authoritative parenting style, with high control and support while maintaining emotional connectedness could be a protective influence preventing NSSI onset. Parents have the ability to moderate the effects of bullying in a way that may prevent NSSI as a coping method. Undefined and uninvolved parenting styles (lacking these protective factors) produce adolescent risk behaviors, which are more likely to include self-injury. One of the first studies to indicate significant differences in deliberate self-harm vs. suicidal participants was one completed by Martin and Waite (1994), which indicates that self-harmers who perceived their parents as more controlling and less caring than their non-self-injuring peers had three times more risk for NSSI than those perceiving ideal parenting. There are clear differences between non-self-harming adolescents and those who engaged in self-harm. These differences can be evident for inconsistent parental relationships that are controlling and cold, but also for those relationships that are weak and extremely warm (Burešová et al., 2015). Adjusting extreme parenting styles can assist in reducing self-injuring behaviors, which in turn, will reduce parental stress (Miller et al., 2007). Hence, protective factors include those caregiving relationships with a consistent, warm, and open parenting style that adjusts structure and boundaries accordingly. Additionally, even if the parenting style is lacking, perceived parental support and connectedness with the child can serve as protective (Claes et al., 2015; Taliaferro & Muehlenkamp, 2017).

Family stressors

Interpersonal correlates for NSSI are also evident in families composed of single or divorced parents. This suggests that a disruption in the family system or parental stress could pose a risk for the development of NSSI behaviors (Burešová et al., 2015). When seeking to understand those who engage in NSSI, researchers have indicated that a significant increase in the quality of the father-child relationship may be protective (Hilt et al., 2008). This finding and others imply that the roles of specific family members, such as parents, are critical in establishing prevention initiatives, treatment, or maintaining the cessation of NSSI. Additionally, there are other childhood stressors related to the family system that are correlated with self-injury. For instance, the socioeconomic status of the family has been strongly associated with self-injury in adolescence. Individuals from low-SES families who engage in NSSI report being concerned with affording basic necessities (Bureau et al., 2010). Economic stressors can cause emotional distress, especially in the life of a young person who has no ability to control financial situations and often is not developmentally capable of understanding monetary dilemmas. Poor family functioning, dysfunction, and broken family bonds are strongly associated with child and adolescent NSSI. Acts of deliberate self-harm and NSSI are potentially associated with the accumulation of various forms of family distress and negative life events (Baetens et al., 2011). The risk factors and correlates of NSSI in children and adolescents are similar in many aspects, but the toll that these factors take on the psychosocial development of a young person differentiates them. Developmental age and cognitive stage, in combination with environmental factors, can serve to be protective with regard to the onset of NSSI. Those who engage in NSSI as children typically lack abstract and logical thinking, and they are not able to disassociate negative events happening within the family from themselves. Children will usually overemphasize their role in the events (Shaw, 2000), which can influence harmful behaviors.

Bullying and victimization

Research examining Integrated Motivational-Volitional Theory (IMV) (O'Connor, 2011) has demonstrated that interpersonal negative life events can be internalized as humiliating or defeating, leading to feelings of entrapment and possible suicidal ideation and attempts. Within the IMV framework, increased capability for suicide (e.g., increased pain threshold or NSSI) amplifies the risk for suicidal ideation and attempts. Interpersonal challenges can support the motivation to turn ideations toward suicide attempts. Lack of social relationships and support, bullying, and isolation are all examples of other interpersonal risk factors that may cause children, teens, and adults to begin or continue to engage in self-injury. Bullying (Claes et al., 2015) and peer exposure to NSSI (Deliberto & Nock, 2008) are important social risk factors for clinicians to consider. When peers observe each other using NSSI as an effective means of coping, social contagion can occur (Jarvi et al., 2013). Students who are both bullied and bullies are at a greater risk for both mental health and behavior problems (Centers for Disease Control, 2017). The National Center for Educational Statistics (2016) estimates that more than 20.8% of students in K–12 settings are bullied. Being a bully is associated with a series of activities that are viewed as delinquent (e.g., physical fights, weapons, theft, and drug use and abuse; Álvarez-García et al., 2015). These experiences could cause youth to become accustomed to the feelings associated with fear and pain. Impulsive and unemotional traits are higher, or more likely evident, for those who bully others. These traits are also connected with risk-taking (Crone et al., 2016), which makes impulsive bullies more likely to engage in NSSI behaviors and suicidal ideation. Notably, physical bullying places adolescents and adults in situations where they are physically injured, thus allowing the bullies to experience physical pain that they do not have to inflict upon themselves. Going into a bullying situation with a desire for or indifference toward injury is a form of indirect NSSI. Exposure to and conditioning through these types of provoked and painful experiences can indirectly build capability for suicide.

Peer victimization is also a strong predictor of NSSI (Bakken & Gunter, 2012). Young people may self-injure as a plea for help or attention, as a form of self-punishment, or for stress relief associated with peer victimization (Nock, 2010). Additional studies specifically show peer victimization and bully perpetration as strongly correlated with NSSI, especially in younger children (Claes et al., 2015; van Geel et al., 2015). A proposed explanation is that children of this age lack the coping skills to address peer victimization, thus leading them to report bullying in combination with NSSI more frequently. The initial onset for NSSI behaviors is typically between the ages of 13 and 15, with another onset peak between the ages of 17 and 24 (Lofthouse & Yager-Schweller, 2009; Whitlock et al., 2006). These periods of onset could be explained by educational transitions typical during these times. Chickering and Reisser (1993) propose that young people perceive the most stress during transitional periods. This theory may also hold true for young children during transitions between primary and secondary educational settings. Prevention programming for younger children implemented during this developmental period could serve to increase support and perhaps prevent engagement in self-injurious behaviors. Lack of social support is a significant predictor of NSSI onset, maintenance, severity, and future engagement. Support from teachers, parents, guardians, and other critical adult figures is protective for children (Taliaferro & Muehlenkamp, 2017). School programming and a protocol designed to address NSSI is essential, even in elementary settings. Additionally, avoidance of punitive responses to children and teens engaging in NSSI will assist in any process design to decrease the behavior. The presence of support from non-parental adults can create a more optimal environment to facilitate termination of the behavior, which is why when younger children hit developmental milestones (psychosocial and cognitive transitions), adult involvement is protective and potentially crucial (Rotolone & Martin, 2012).

Intrapersonal factors

When examining interpersonal risk factors for NSSI in adults, many of the same factors that were present in childhood and adolescence are relevant. Early childhood or adolescent history of NSSI and continued engagement into young adulthood are the strongest risk factors for NSSI in adults (Fox et al., 2015). Interpersonal risk factors are also prevalent well into adulthood. Self-injurers are much more likely than non-injurers to have a family history of mental health issues, alcoholism, drug abuse, violence, past sexual abuse, and suicidal ideation. Additional challenges with romantic partners, potentially linked to attachment issues from childhood, could affect emotional regulation capacity in adult romantic relationships, creating unhealthy attachment in the relationship and use of NSSI as a means to cope with emergent emotional dysregulation (Crowell et al., 2009). Similar to the cases of children and adolescents, family support is identified as the most prominent predictor of NSSI cessation and is considered a protective factor (Tatnell et al., 2014), and absence of support is most significantly related to the onset of NSSI in adulthood (Baetens et al., 2014). However, most research on associations between NSSI and family factors is deficient in defining a clear conceptual model of family functioning. For older adult and elderly populations, intrapersonal risk factors include social isolation, bereavement or loss, and physical illness.

History

According to numerous studies, prior history of NSSI is the strongest identified risk factor for future suicide attempts, and suicidal ideation is a risk factor for NSSI. Franklin et al. (2017) recently supported these findings, indicating that suicidal thoughts and self-injury are likely risk factors for suicide attempts and possible death. This outcome aligns with the research suggesting NSSI is the single best predictor of eventual suicide (Beauchaine et al., 2015). Within the elderly population, those who self-injure are found to be at 67 times greater risk for committing suicide than elderly individuals who do not engage in NSSI. Additionally, 90% of the elderly population that is depressed and engaging in self-harm commit suicide (Merrill & Owens, 1990; Murphy et al., 2012). This finding is startling. Suicidal thoughts, behaviors, and self-injury in the elderly population need clear and a thorough assessment for risk, due to the interconnectedness of these behaviors.

While these intrapersonal factors can be worked on in therapy, some of the interpersonal factors (such as sexual abuse, past violence, bullying) that may have caused the intrapersonal factors and feeling states cannot be directly changed. It is important to assume that the current intrapersonal factors that contributed to the start and continuance of NSSI are amenable to change and thus may contribute to the intervention, treatment, and prevention of future NSSI. NSSI is noted in the literature as a way to cope with negative feeling states that cause emotional turmoil or dysregulation (Nock, 2010). Emotional regulation theories of NSSI work under the premise that those who utilize NSSI have high levels of emotion dysregulation and these feelings cause people to initiate engagement in NSSI to improve their mood (Franklin et al., 2017). People currently engaging in NSSI are more likely than those with a history of NSSI to articulate the role of NSSI as a way to control negative affect. They also have less impulse control and have higher emotional suppression (Andrews et al., 2013). This implies that the period to assesses NSSI is critical, as is the choice of instrumentation.

Hopelessness and self-esteem

One of the strongest intrapersonal risk factors for NSSI is hopelessness, which is also a significant risk factor for suicidal ideation and behavior. Suicidal thoughts often stem from hopelessness (Fox et al., 2015) and low self-esteem. Low self-esteem is of the utmost importance because if it is tied to past and current NSSI behavior, it can also predict the risk for suicidal behaviors. Those who have greater amounts of self-criticism and negative self-talk typically have lower levels of self-esteem. Ross et al. (2009) found that those engaging in NSSI had greater body dissatisfaction and a sense of ineffectiveness. This aligns with the factor that engagement in NSSI is often found in those with an eating disorder. Along the same lines, negative self-concept is associated with NSSI engagement, which supports the theory that NSSI could be used as a method to alleviate these negative emotions and as a form of self-punishment (Ross et al., 2009). This is important for clinicians working with current self-injurers and those with a history of self-injury. Understanding correlates for current vs. past NSSI is essential to determining the risk assessment and treatment of NSSI in clients. Those with low self-esteem use the self-injury as a motive for self-punishment, and to cope with feelings of shame (Sornberger et al., 2012). Those who are shame prone may utilize NSSI to manage shame-triggering stressors. Intrapersonal functions are used to regulate, express, and change emotional states, and shame is an important psychological state that is managed and changed through NSSI (Mahtani et al., 2018). The link between shame and NSSI again sheds light on the high co-occurrence of NSSI and internalizing disorders (e.g., mood and eating disorders).

Risky behaviors

Many studies show that those engaging in NSSI also smoke cigarettes, use drugs, or engage in other health-risk behaviors, such as binging, purging, poor body image, and unhealthy dating relationships (Hilt et al., 2008). While this information assists clinicians when examining risk factors for NSSI, it remains unclear if these correlates are predictors or outcomes of NSSI behaviors or simply co-exist due to underlying contextual issues. This is important to consider when working with those who engage in NSSI. Behaviors that are possible consequences of NSSI also have the potential to be corrected if there is a cessation of the NSSI behavior. Conversely, if something is a precursor or risk factor (e.g., binge eating), finding a way to address that factor (the disordered eating) will assist in the cessation of the NSSI behavior. To further understand the phenomenology of NSSI, it will be important for future research to examine a broad age range in larger samples of children and adolescents, which follows them over time, to determine when each of these health risk behaviors develops in relation to the others.

Biological concerns

Findings from neurobiological studies have begun to make connections between NSSI and altered patterns in the brain (specifically the hypothalamic-pituitary-adrenal [HPA] axis) that serve as structures to assist in coping with stressful situations. This change indicates a difference in the processing of emotional pain, which would put some at greater risk for repeat NSSI (Reichl et al., 2016). The genetic background of those who engage in self-injury reveals an association with the genes involved in serotonergic neurotransmission (Hankin et al., 2011). Serotonin is a neurotransmitter in the brain involved in mood regulation, social behavior, appetite, digestion, sleep, sexual function, and memory. Results from fMRI studies found those who engage in NSSI have hyperarousal of limbic structures (such as the amygdala and the anterior cingulate cortex [ACC]) (Plener et al., 2012), which puts them at a higher risk for engaging in NSSI. ACC structures have been linked to anxiety, impulse control, and other higher cognitive functions in addition to autonomic functions such as blood pressure regulation. The hyperarousal of these brain structures decreases after individuals with a history of NSSI engage in painful stimulus or self-injury. Additionally, the hyperarousal is reduced through imagining an act of NSSI (Kraus et al., 2010), which poses a great deal of promise in treatment strategies.

Novelty- and sensation-seeking increase significantly during puberty, which is a time period when the ability to self-regulate is low and not fully developed. This intrapersonal factor of puberty combined with other psychosocial facets can cause detrimental consequences for those at risk of engaging in NSSI and lifetime self-injurers. Evidence suggests that there is a connection between impulsive behaviors and a lack of serotonin, but NSSI is characteristically not an impulsive behavior, which supports the notion that NSSI is utilized, in part, due to an issue with serotonergic neurotransmission. It is possible that those with serotonin deficiency, or insufficient stress response, are more likely to engage in NSSI to compensate for emotional regulatory systems (Groschwitz & Plener, 2012).

Risk factors related to diversity

Many societal and cultural issues differentially intersect to affect certain groups, placing some at greater risk for NSSI. Currently, research shows females report higher rates of NSSI and may be at a slightly higher risk for certain methods of NSSI than their male counterparts (Sornberger et al., 2012). It is not clear if this difference is due to biological and/or cultural messages or if females are just more likely to report their self-injury. Until recently, much of the literature did not explore NSSI in males. Additionally, there are findings that indicate clinicians may inaccurately conceptualize and assess males who self-injure (Healey et al., 2010), which may better explain why females report higher rates or why female self-injury is more likely to be captured in clinical studies. Several recent studies have also found no significant difference between male and female NSSI when accounting for multiple methods of engaging in the behavior (beyond cutting). Adolescents cope with the development of complex relational emotions and increasingly demanding educational challenges; thus, they are more likely to turn to NSSI to regulate their emotional experience when their environment is not supportive or affirming. Additionally, elderly males are at an increased risk for deliberate self-harm potentially due to patriarchal and gender role stereotypes that can negatively influence perceptions of self. There is often a loss of meaning during transitions to retirement, loss of physical and sexual functioning, and loss of perceived status and power.

It is well known that Caucasian individuals tend to be more likely to report a history of NSSI (Muehlenkamp & Gutierrez, 2007), though this does not imply additional risk. Croyle (2007) postulated that Hispanic men's adherence to traditional roles and values from Mexican culture serves as a protective factor against NSSI in this cultural group. This example highlights how ethnic or cultural connectedness can be protective. Several studies show certain cultural groups report NSSI more frequently than others do. For example, Wester & Trepal (2015) found African American and Asian American college students to be significantly less likely to participate in NSSI than Caucasian, Hispanic, and Multiracial/Other students. They hypothesize that a sense of belonging, as opposed to ethnic identity, decreases engagement in NSSI in general for most racial groups. This sense of belonging may explain the differences in NSSI prevalence noted across racial and ethnic groups. Older adults with low SES, traditional cultural beliefs, and more physical illnesses are also at higher risk due to less access to services as they age. Lesbian, gay, and bisexual (LGB) youth have been shown to be a subgroup particularly affected by self-harming behaviors (Deliberto & Nock, 2008), and they experience a greater risk for NSSI and suicide. Though very few studies examine the risk for trans youth, there has been some evidence of increased risk for suicidal ideation and self-harm. Sexual minority youth have up to eight times greater prevalence of NSSI compared to their heterosexual peers (Taliaferro & Muehlenkamp, 2017). Hatzenbuehler's psychological mediation framework (2009) attempts to describe how sexual minorities experience higher levels of stress as a result of stigma. This stigma places sexual minorities at a higher risk of emotional dysregulation and interpersonal difficulties. Hence, stigma may mediate or moderate the relationship found between sexual minority stress and related psychopathology, or in this case NSSI. Culture and diversity factors related to NSSI are further explored in Chapter 6.

Ecological conceptualization

Understanding the person plus environment fit can sometimes be complex, especially given all of the factors and considerations reviewed in this chapter. Neufeld and colleagues (2006) proposed a model for understanding the person-environment interaction through system engagement that may facilitate a growth-promotion in conceptualizing client need. They suggest perceiving client need through person-environment engagement, including three components: (1) negotiation, (2) participation, and (3) evaluation. Negotiation involves balancing environmental factors like physical and social resources and stressors with personal strengths and limitations. Once negotiation occurs, one is able to participate and then evaluate that participation to assess personal achievement and desired environmental enhancements at home, school, and work. Further, Williams, McMahon, and Goodman (2015) suggested clinicians utilize an eco-webbing process model to assist in the development of treatment plans consistent with person-environment interaction concepts. In this three-phase process, clinicians think about factors contributing to the client's behavior on multiple system levels (see Appendix F for Bronfenbrenner's worksheet), consider the most salient themes that may align with their role as counselors and the counseling process, and then reflect on the decisions made and how they will inform treatment. Reflecting on the intra- and interpersonal context of a client's life can assist clinicians in developing appropriate treatment plans and monitoring treatment progress from a contextual perspective. While we, and other scholars, recommend this process for use with all clients as a way of identifying risk and protective factors, needs, strengths, and limitations, its use is particularly important in working with high-risk individuals, like those engaging in non-suicidal self-injury.

At this point, you should have reviewed all of the interpersonal and intrapersonal risk factors, correlates, precursors, and protective factors in each of the cases presented in prior chapters. Table 4.1 contains each of the cases and the risk and protective factors that might be typical, given the information provided. Many of the factors listed have been found to be directly associated with NSSI and some are indirectly associated (i.e., linked to related mental health concerns and/or suicidal ideation).

Table 4.1 Potential risk and protective factors in each case study

Case	*Risk factor/correlate*	*Protective factor*
Jenny	• Family stressors • Separating parents • Differing parenting styles between mom and dad • Poor coping skills • Multiple heritage • Confusing home life issues between mom and dad	• Performs well in school • Well-liked by peer groups • Good attachment with parents • Involved with extracurricular activities • Multiple heritage
Sam	• Lack of parental figure in the home • Lack of friends and peer groups • Bullied at school • Lots of alone time • Lack of clear and consistent parenting style (indulgent parenting style) • Behavioral issues at school and unsupportive school environment • Peers are supportive of his NSSI behaviors • Educational transition to middle school	• A supportive mother who wants to help • Still performing adequately in school • A few friends
Emma	• Past trauma, sexual abuse • Parental attachment is likely poor • No male role model or positive male relationships • Disruptive in school and dropping grades from age 15 on • History of suicide in the family • Past history of suicidal ideations • Friends that engage in NSSI • About to transition to college or the world of work post-high school graduation	• Supportive grandmother • She can utilize less severe methods of NSSI to cope • Cultural identity and heritage • Open with her counselor and willing to engage in treatment • Authoritative parenting style

(*Continued*)

Table 4.1 (Continued) Potential risk and protective factors in each case study

Case	*Risk factor/correlate*	*Protective factor*
Rick	• Lack of attachment with mother • Disruptive behavior and poor grades in school • Diagnosis of ODD and ADD • Authoritarian parenting style • Recent transition to high school	• Supportive father and grandmother • Supportive relationship • School is supportive and trying to help • Possible spiritual beliefs and connectedness
Charlotte	• Bisexual, non-binary status • History of sexual abuse • Recent transition to college and living on her own in a dorm • Possible eating-disordered behavior • Ill family member • History of depression and isolation	• Semi-supportive mother and stepfather • Willing to engage in therapy • Intelligent • Peer relationships • A healthy intimate relationship • Authoritative parenting style
Jimmy	• History of substance and narcotics abuse • History of lifetime NSSI • History of suicide attempts • Current suicidal ideation • Low insight and willingness to seek support • Gender-related conflict present	• A supportive relationship with his partner • Connectedness to racial and cultural identity
Rhonda	• Domestic violence survivor • Transition into the work force • History of NSSI • Anxiety and fear as a result of past domestic abuse	• Children • Engagement in counseling and willingness to seek support • Peer support
Dean	• Lifetime history of NSSI • Identifies as a gay male • Loss of support system • Physical health issues • Non-compliant with medications	• Spiritual/religious connection • Willing to engage in counseling and seek help • Friends for support • Willing to engage in therapy

TEXTBOX 4.1 REFLECTING ON SIGNIFICANCE AND IMPACT OF RISK AND PROTECTIVE FACTORS

Now that you have reviewed the extensive list of risk and protective factors in regard to NSSI, there are some important things to keep in mind when considering application of this information in practice.

Many risk and protective factors are associated with multiple outcomes. That is, they are important influences in many mental health and developmental concerns. These factors are a great place to start when assessing individuals to determine appropriate avenues for care. For example, poor parental attachment is a risk factor NSSI, but also for attachment disorders, substance abuse and use disorders, anxiety disorders, many personality disorders and styles, engaging in unhealthy relationships, and so on. We cannot jump to conclusions that some of these broad factors are going to cause NSSI in clients, as relationships can exists without causality.

Not all risk and protective factors are equivalent. Some risk and protective factors are more significant than others. For example, it is likely that adolescents who self-injure also have a friend who does. Having friends who engage in self-injury is an important risk factor (Jarvi et al., 2013), potentially more so than simply having the means (i.e., razors or sharp objects) readily available. It's important to consider the comparative importance of each risk and protective factor because this will assist you in prioritizing clinical attention.

The more risk factors present, the greater the possibility they will engage in the behavior. Conversely, the more protective factors or assets they have, the less likely they are to engage in an associated destructive behavior (CDC, 2018). For example, if you eat a diet high in cholesterol, don't exercise, are overweight, have high blood pressure, and a family history of heart disease, it's much more probable that you will have a heart attack than if you have the single risk factor of being overweight.

REFERENCES

Álvarez-García, D., García, T., & Núñez, J.C. (2015). Predictors of school bullying perpetration in adolescence: A systematic review. *Aggression and Violent Behavior*, 23, 126–136. doi:10.1016/j.avb.2015.05.007

Andrews, T., Martin, G., Hasking, P., & Page, A. (2013). Predictors of continuation and cessation of nonsuicidal self-injury. *Journal of Adolescent Health*, 53(1), 40–46. doi:10.1016/j.jadohealth.2013.01.009

Arbuthnott, A.E., & Lewis, S.P. (2015). Parents of youth who self-injure: A review of the literature and implications for mental health professionals. *Child and Adolescent Psychiatry and Mental Health*, 9(1), 35. doi:10.1186/s13034-015-0066-3

Baetens, I., Claes, L., Muehlenkamp, J., Grietens, H., & Onghena, P. (2011). Non-suicidal and suicidal self-injurious behavior among Flemish adolescents: A web-survey. *Archives of Suicide Research*, 15(1), 56–67. doi:10.1080/13811118.2011.540467

Baetens, I., Claes, L., Martin, G., Onghena, P., Grietens, H., Van Leeuwen, K., … Griffith, J.W. (2014). Is nonsuicidal selfinjury associated with parenting and family factors? *The Journal of Early Adolescence*, 34, 387–405. doi:10.1177/0272431613494006

Baetens, I., Claes, L., Muehlenkamp, J., Grietens, H., & Onghena, P. (2012). Differences in psychological symptoms and self-competencies in non-suicidal self-injurious Flemish adolescents. *Journal of Adolescence*, 35(3), 753–759. doi:10.1016/j.adolescence.2011.11.001

Bakken, N.W., & Gunter, W.D. (2012). Self-cutting and suicidal ideation among adolescents: Gender differences in the causes and correlates of self-injury. *Deviant Behavior*, 33(5), 339–356. doi:10.1080/01639625.2011.584054

Beauchaine, T.P., Crowell, S.E., & Hsiao, R.C. (2015). Post-dexamethasone cortisol, self-inflicted injury, and suicidal ideation among depressed adolescent girls. *Journal of Abnormal Child Psychology*, 43(4), 619–632. doi:10.1007/s10802-014-9933-2

Bowlby, J. (1973). *Attachment and Loss* (vol. 2). New York, NY: Basic Books.

Bureau, J.F., Martin, J., Freynet, N., Poirier, A.A., Lafontaine, M.F., & Cloutier, P. (2010). Perceived dimensions of parenting and non-suicidal self-injury in young adults. *Journal of Youth and Adolescence*, 39(5), 484–494. doi:10.1007/s10964-009-9470-4

Burešová, I., Bartošová, K., & Čerňák, M. (2015). Connection between parenting styles and self-harm in adolescence. *Procedia-Social and Behavioral Sciences*, 171, 1106–1113. doi:10.1016/j.sbspro.2015.01.272

Centers for Disease Control and Prevention. (2017). *Bullying*. Retrieved January 2, 2017 from https://www.cdc.gov/violenceprevention/youthviolence/bullyingresearch/index.html

Centers for Disease Control and Prevention. (2018). Risk and protective factors. Retrieved July 19, 2019 from https://www.cdc.gov/violenceprevention/suicide/riskprotectivefactors.html

Chickering, A.W., & Reisser, L. (1993). *Education and Identity. The Jossey-Bass Higher and Adult Education Series*. San Francisco, CA: Jossey-Bass Inc.

Claes, L., Luyckx, K., Baetens, I., Van de Ven, M., & Witteman, C. (2015). Bullying and victimization, depressive mood, and non-suicidal self-injury in adolescents: The moderating role of parental support. *Journal of Child and Family Studies*, 24(11), 3363–3371. doi:10.1007/s10826-015-0138-2

Crone, E.A., van Duijvenvoorde, A.C., & Peper, J.S. (2016). Annual Research Review: Neural contributions to risk-taking in adolescence–developmental changes and individual differences. *Journal of Child Psychology and Psychiatry*, 57(3), 353–368. doi:10.1111/jcpp.12502

Crowell, S.E., Beauchaine, T.P., & Linehan, M.M. (2009). A biosocial developmental model of borderline personality: Elaborating and extending Linehan's theory. *Psychological Bulletin*, 135, 495–510. doi:10.1037/a0015616

Croyle, K. (2007). Self-harm experiences among Hispanic and non-Hispanic White young adults. *Hispanic Journal of Behavioral Sciences*, 29, 242–253. doi:10.1177/0739986307299452

Deliberto, T.L., & Nock, M.K. (2008). An exploratory study of correlates, onset, and offset of non-suicidal self-injury. *Archives of Suicide Research*, 12(3), 219–231. doi:10.1080/13811110802101096

Dunn, V.J., Abbott, R.A., Croudace, T.J., Wilkinson, P., Jones, P.B., Herbert, J., & Goodyer, I.M. (2011). Profiles of family-focused adverse experiences through childhood and early adolescence: The ROOTS project a community investigation of adolescent mental health. *BMC Psychiatry*, 11(1), 109. doi:10.1186/1471-244x-11-109

Fox, K.R., Franklin, J.C., Ribeiro, J.D., Kleiman, E.M., Bentley, K.H., & Nock, M.K. (2015). Meta-analysis of risk factors for nonsuicidal self-injury. *Clinical Psychology Review*, 42, 156–167. doi:10.1016/j.cpr.2015.09.002

Franklin, J.C., Ribeiro, J.D., Fox, K.R., Bentley, K.H., Kleiman, E.M., Huang, X., … & Nock, M.K. (2017). Risk factors for suicidal thoughts and behaviors: A meta-analysis of 50 years of research. *Psychological Bulletin*, 143(2), 187. doi:10.1037/bul0000084

Groschwiz, R.C. & Plener, P.L. (2012). The neurobiology of Non-Suicidal Self-Injury (NSSI): A review. *Suicidology Online*, 3, 24–32.

Hankin, B.L., Barrocas, A.L., Jennes, J., Oppenheimer, C.W., Badanes, L.S., Abela, J.R., Young, J., & Smolen, A. (2011). Association between 5-HTTLPR and borderline personality disorder traits among youth. *Journal of Clinical Child & Adolescent* Psychology, 40, 572–585. doi:10.3389/fpsyt.2011.00006

Hatzenbuehler, M.L. (2009). How does sexual minority stigma "get under the skin"? A psychological mediation framework. *Psychological Bulletin*, 135(5), 707. doi:10.1037/a0016441

Hay, C., & Meldrum, R. (2010). Bullying victimization and adolescent self-harm: Testing hypotheses from general strain theory. *Journal of Youth and Adolescence*, 39(5), 446–459. doi:10.1007/s10964-009-9502-0

Healey, A., Trepal, H., & Emelianchik-Key, K. (2010). Nonsuicidal self-injury: Examining the relationship between diagnosis and gender. *Journal of Mental Health Counseling*, 32(4), 324–341. doi:10.17744/mehc.32.4.366740506r458202

Hilt, L.M., Nock, M.K., Lloyd-Richardson, E.E., & Prinstein, M.J. (2008). Longitudinal study of nonsuicidal self-injury among young adolescents: Rates, correlates, and preliminary test of an interpersonal model. *The Journal of Early Adolescence*, 28(3), 455–469. doi:10.1177/0272431608316604

James, K.M., & Gibb, B.E. (2019). Maternal criticism and non-suicidal self-injury in school-aged children. *Psychiatry Research*, 273, 89–93. doi:10.1016/j.psychres.2019.01.019

Jarvi, S., Jackson, B., Swenson, L., & Crawford, H. (2013). The impact of social contagion on non-suicidal self-injury: A review of the literature. *Archives of Suicide Research*, 17(1), 1–19. doi:10.1080/13811118.2013.748404

Kena, G., Hussar, W., McFarland, J., de Brey, C., Musu-Gillette, L., Wang, X., … & Barmer, A. (2016). The Condition of Education 2016. NCES 2016–144. *National Center for Education Statistics*. Retrieved from https://nces.ed.gov/pubs2016/2016144.pdf

Kokaliari, E.D. (2014). An exploratory study of the nature and extent of nonsuicidal self-injury among college women. *International Journal of Population Research*, 2014. doi:10.1155/2014/879269

Kraemer, H.C., Kazdin, A.E., Offord, D.R., Kessler, R.C., Jensen, P.S., & Kupfer, D.J. (1997). Coming to terms with the terms of risk. *Archives of General Psychiatry*, 54(4), 337–343. doi:10.1001/archpsyc.1997.01830160065009

Kraus, A., Valerius, G., Seifritz, E., Ruf, M., Bremner, J.D., Bohus, M., & Schmahl, C. (2010). Script-driven imagery of self-injurious behaviour in patients with borderline personality disorder: A pilot FMRI study. *Acta Psychiatrica Scandinavica*, 121, 41–51. doi:10.1111/j.1600-0447.2009.01417.x

Lofthouse, N., & Yager-Schweller, J. (2009). Nonsuicidal self-injury and suicide risk among adolescents. *Current Opinion in Pediatrics*, 21(5), 641–645. doi:10.1097/mop.0b013e3283306825

Mahtani, S., Melvin, G.A., & Hasking, P. (2018). Shame proneness, shame coping, and functions of nonsuicidal self-injury (NSSI) among emerging adults: A developmental analysis. *Emerging Adulthood*, 6(3), 159–171. doi:10.1177/2167696817711350

Martin, G., & Waite, S. (1994). Parental bonding and vulnerability to adolescent suicide. *Acta Psychiatrica Scandinavica*, 89(4), 246–254. doi:10.1111/j.1600-0447.1994.tb01509.x

Merrill, J., & Owens, J. (1990). Age and attempted suicide. *Acta Psychiatrica Scandinavica*, 82(5), 385–388. doi:10.1111/j.1600-0447.1990.tb01407.x

Miller, A.L., Rathus, J.H., & Linehan, M.M. (2007). *Dialectical Behavior with Suicidal Adolescents*. New York, NY: The Guildford Press. doi:10.5617/suicidologi.1788

Muehlenkamp, J.J., & Gutierrez, P.M. (2007). Risk for suicide attempts among adolescents who engage in non-suicidal self-injury. *Archives of Suicide Research*, 11(1), 69–82. doi:10.1080/13811110600992902

Murphy, E., Kapur, N., Webb, R., Purandare, N., Hawton, K., Bergen, H., Waters, K., & Cooper, J. (2012). Risk factors for repetition and suicide following self-harm in older adults: Multicentre cohort study. *British Journal of Psychiatry*, 200(5), 399–404. doi:10.1192/bjp.bp.111.094177

Neufeld, J.E., Rasmussen, H.N., Lopez, S.J., Ryder, J.A., Magyar-Moe, J.L., Ford, A.I., ... Bouwkamp, J.C. (2006). The engagement model of person-environment interaction. *The Counseling Psychologist*, 34(2), 245–259. doi:10.1177/0011000005281319

Nock, M.K. (2010). Self-injury. *Annual Review of Clinical Psychology*, 6, 339–363. doi:10.1146/annurev.clinpsy.121208.131258

O'Connor, R.C. (2011). The integrated motivational-volitional model of suicidal behavior. *Crisis* 32(6), 295–298. doi:10.1027/0227-5910/a000120

Plener, P.L., Bubalo, N., Fladung, A.K., Ludolph, A.G., & Lulé, D. (2012). Prone to excitement: Adolescent females with non-suicidal self-injury (NSSI) show altered cortical pattern to emotional and NSS-related material. *Psychiatry Research: Neuroimaging*, 203(2–3), 146–152. doi:10.1016/j.pscychresns.2011.12.012

Polk, E. & Liss, M. (2007). Psychological characteristics of self-injurious behaviour. *Personality and Individual Differences*, 43, 567–577. doi:10.1016/j.paid.2007.01.003

Reichl, C., Heyer, A., Brunner, R., Parzer, P., Völker, J.M., Resch, F., & Kaess, M. (2016). Hypothalamic-pituitary-adrenal axis, childhood adversity and adolescent nonsuicidal self-injury. *Psychoneuroendocrinology*, 74, 203–211. doi:10.1016/j.psyneuen.2016.09.011

Ross, S., Heath, N.L., & Toste, J.R. (2009). Non-suicidal self-injury and eating pathology in high school students. *American Journal of Orthopsychiatry*, 79(1), 83–92. doi:10.1037/a0014826

Rotolone, C., & Martin, G. (2012). Giving up self-injury: A comparison of everyday social and personal resources in past versus current self-injurers. *Archives of Suicide Research*, 16(2), 147–158. doi:10.1080/13811118.2012.667333

Serafini, G., Canepa, G., Adavastro, G., Nebbia, J., Belvederi Murri, M., Erbuto, D., ... & Amore, M. (2017). The relationship between childhood maltreatment and non-suicidal self-injury: A systematic review. *Frontiers in Psychiatry*, 8, 149. doi:10.3389/fpsyt.2017.00149

Shaw, J.A. (2000). Children, adolescents, and trauma. *Psychiatric Quarterly*, 71, 227–243. doi:10.1023/a:1004630127000

Snyder, C.R., & Lopez, S.J. (Eds.). (2001). *Handbook of Positive Psychology*. New York, NY: Oxford University Press. doi:10.1093/oxfordhb/9780195187243.001.0001

Sornberger, M.J., Heath, N.L., Toste, J.R., & McLouth, R. (2012). Nonsuicidal self-injury and gender: Patterns of prevalence, methods, and locations among adolescents. *Suicide and Life-Threatening Behavior*, 42(3), 266–278. doi:10.1111/j.1943-278x.2012.0088.x

Taliaferro, L.A., & Muehlenkamp, J.J. (2017). Nonsuicidal self-injury and suicidality among sexual minority youth: Risk factors and protective connectedness factors. *Academic Pediatrics*, 17(7), 715–722. doi:10.1016/j.acap.2016.11.002

Tatnell, R., Kelada, L., Hasking, P., & Martin, G. (2014). Longitudinal analysis of adolescent NSSI: The role of intrapersonal and interpersonal factors. *Journal of Abnormal Child Psychology*, 42(6), 885–896. doi:10.1007/s10802-013-9837-6

van Geel, M., Goemans, A., & Vedder, P. (2015). A meta-analysis on the relation between peer victimization and adolescent non-suicidal self-injury. *Psychiatry Research*, 230(2), 364–368. doi:10.1016/j.psychres.2015.09.017

van Harmelen, A.L., Gibson, J.L., St Clair, M.C., Owens, M., Brodbeck, J., Dunn, V., ... & Goodyer, I.M. (2016). Friendships and family support reduce subsequent depressive symptoms in at-risk adolescents. *PLOS ONE*, 11(5), e0153715. doi:10.1371/journal.pone.0153715

Wedig, M.M., & Nock, M.K. (2007). Parental expressed emotion and adolescent self-injury. *Journal of the American Academy of Child & Adolescent Psychiatry*, 46(9), 1171–1178. doi:10.1097/chi.0b013e3180ca9aaf

Wester, K.L., & Trepal, H.C. (2015). Nonsuicidal self-injury: Exploring the connection among race, ethnic identity, and ethnic belonging. *Journal of College Student Development*, 56(2), 127–139. doi:10.1353/csd.2015.0013

West, M., Rose, M.S., Spreng, S., Sheldon-Keller, A., & Adam, K. (1998). Adolescent attachment questionnaire: A brief assessment of attachment in adolescence. *Journal of Youth and Adolescence*, 27(5), 661–673. doi:10.1023/a:1022891225542

Williams, J.M., McMahon, H.G., & Goodman, R.D. (2015). Eco-webbing: A teaching strategy to facilitate critical consciousness and agency. *Counselor Education and Supervision*, 54(2), 82–97. doi:10.1002/ceas.12006

Whitlock, J., Eckenrode, J., & Silverman, D. (2006). Self-injurious behaviors in a college population. *Pediatrics*, 117(6), 1939–1948. doi:10.1542/peds.2005-2543

Yates, T.M., Carlson, E.A., & Egeland, B. (2008). A prospective study of child maltreatment and self-injurious behavior in a community sample. *Development and Psychopathology*, 20(2), 651–671. doi:10.1017/s0954579408000321

You, J., & Leung, F. (2012). The role of depressive symptoms, family invalidation and behavioral impulsivity in the occurrence and repetition of non-suicidal self-injury in Chinese adolescents: A 2-year follow-up study. *Journal of Adolescence*, 35(2), 389–395. doi:10.1016/j.adolescence.2011.07.020

5 Assessment and diagnosis

Kelly Emelianchik-Key

Non-suicidal self-injury can be difficult to conceptualize. As you may have noticed, no two cases are alike, and much of the research that has been done previously only focuses on small and non-diverse samples. Additionally, it can be challenging to sort through research to find studies that focus on clinical and non-clinical populations. To fully understand the problem of NSSI, we must first conceptualize NSSI in a way that considers diversity, and that does not put everyone into a distinct box or category. As you will start to notice, NSSI is unique and conceptualizing clients can be challenging since there is still so much information that is unknown about NSSI.

Defining self-injury

To begin, let's review the definition of self-injury. NSSI is the intentional and deliberate harm of a person's own body without an attempt to die (Nock, 2010). It is an umbrella term that includes self-injury and self-mutilation. Harm behaviors can include but are not limited to: cutting, burning, hitting, punching, banging, biting, pinching and pulling the skin, and severe scratching. The actions do not include those considered socially sanctioned (e.g., tattoos or piercings) or those behaviors that are a result of another better-explained mental or physical impairment. The most common locations for self-injuries are on the arms, stomach, thighs, hands, calves, ankles, and wrists. The key factor to remember when examining NSSI is that the attempt to die should not be present for the client when engaging in the behavior. Most often, the NSSI is understood in the literature as a coping mechanism or way of controlling emotions, thoughts, and feelings that are unwanted (Nock, 2010). Even though the intent to die is not present at the time of injury, with prolonged and repeated NSSI, suicidality becomes strongly associated with the behavior (Joiner, 2007). NSSI and suicidality can co-exist, but the act of self-injury does not involve the intent to die and can be viewed as a preventative measure taken by the injurer.

Additionally, other severe physical and mental comorbidities are related to NSSI, such as depression, anxiety, eating disorders, substance use disorders, and violent relationships (Nock et al., 2006). Non-suicidal self-injury was added to the *Diagnostic and Statistical Manual of Mental Disorders-5* (DSM-5) as a condition for further study. The DSM-5 uses the following criteria in Table 5.1 to conceptualize self-injury.

Table 5.1 DSM-5 diagnostic criteria for NSSI

A. Intentionally self-inflicting harm to one's body surface knowing that the injury will lead to minor to moderate physical harm and damage, without suicidal intent

B. Intentionally self-injuring the body with the intention that one of the following will result:
   1. Relief from the negative feeling state
   2. Resolve an interpersonal difficulty or struggle
   3. Produce a more calm or positive feeling state

C. Non-suicidal self-injury is associated with one or more of the following:
   1. Interpersonal difficulties or negative feelings or thoughts, such as depression anxiety, tension, anger, generalized distress, or self-criticism occurring in the period immediately before the self-injurious act
   2. There are prior consuming thoughts about the act, and inability to control one's self from engaging in it
   3. When in distress, thoughts of NSSI frequently occur, even if the urge is resisted

D. The behavior is not socially sanctioned (e.g., body piercing, and tattooing) and is not restricted to picking a scab or nail biting (which could classify as another DSM disorder)

E. The NSSI or its consequences cause significant distress or interference in interpersonal functioning or other areas of life

F. The NSSI does not exclusively occur during a psychotic episode, delirium, substance intoxication, or substance withdrawal. Another mental health disorder should not better explain the behavior or medical condition (e.g., psychotic disorder, autism spectrum disorder, intellectual disability, trichotillomania [hair-pulling disorder], excoriation [skin-picking] disorder)

Summary of NSSI disorder diagnostic criterion

The diagnostic criteria noted above are listed in Section III of the DSM-5. This section, "Emerging Measures and Models," refers to the conditions that warrant further study due to the lack of reliability in clinical trials. When assessing self-injury, it is important to keep in mind that the self-injury cannot be accounted for or explained by a diagnosis or the symptom of another diagnosis. For example, if the client has schizophrenia and has auditory delusions that tell them to harm themselves, the schizophrenia would still account for the self-injury. NSSI occurs as a condition within several other diagnoses, such as mood disorders, eating disorders, personality disorders, and substance use disorders. When this co-morbidity occurs, it is referred to as a transdiagnostic behavior (Lofthouse et al., 2008). Many studies examine correlates of NSSI within the context of these other diagnoses, but this practice provides an incomplete picture of NSSI since it can be seen in the absence of other disorders as well. When working with children, diagnoses should always be made with caution, while taking into account that numerous diagnoses cannot be assigned to children under the age of 18 because they are still developing and maturing (American Psychiatric Association, 2013).

Conceptualizing NSSI in children, adolescents, and adults

Currently, there is limited information about self-directed violence in children under the age of 14, which includes both suicide and NSSI. There is also sparse information on how NSSI characteristics develop and progress beyond the age of onset. There is strong evidence showing that children as young as seven years of age are engaging in forms of self-directed violence. A recent study found that 1 in 12 children engaged in NSSI at least once, and 8% of those reporting deliberate self-harm were third graders (Barrocas et al., 2012). Additionally, suicide becomes the second leading cause of death for children at and over the age of 10 (CDC, 2014). As NSSI increases the risk of suicide attempts in children, both behaviors are discussed within the construct of self-directed violence.

Gauging the prevalence of self-harm in children can be challenging since most young children and adolescents who are engaging in harm do not seek help and/or caretakers are unaware of the behavior or how to handle it (Rowe et al., 2014). In the "Cases of Jenny and Sam," their parents are unclear how to handle the self-injury, and they ignore the behaviors for a while to avoid drawing attention to it. The fear of making self-injury worse by bringing attention to it is a common concern among parents. However, when children and teens allow adults to view their scars or injuries, it is often a cry for help and attention. In the cases of Jenny and Sam, they both give their parents glimpses of the self-injuries from time to time. This could be intentional as a way of seeking help and attention. Jenny also chooses to engage in the form of self-injury that cannot be hidden from her parents (hair pulling), which again could be a deliberate and intentional choice in the method of self-injury.

There is currently limited information about self-directed violence in children under the age of 14, which includes both suicide and NSSI. The lack of information is because most self-harm and NSSI information are gathered from school-based surveys (Madge et al., 2008), with little information coming from those who needed medical treatment for their injuries. This said, there is strong evidence that finds children as young as seven years of age are engaging in forms of self-directed violence. Until recently, most of the research that exists with NSSI in young children has stemmed from small inpatient samples. Therefore, it is not uncommon to find a lack of information that provides a clear consensus and evidence base on how to conceptualize and treat young clients who self-injure.

Headbanging, self-biting, scratching with fingernails or other objects, hand mouthing, biting, hair pulling, and punching are some of the common examples of self-injury behaviors in younger children. In the "Case of Jenny" she is an example of a young client who injures in these ways. She began headbanging around age six, and then, eventually, the self-injurious behaviors progressed to hitting herself and hair-pulling. This could be because her stress increased with age, and her parents disregarded the headbanging symptoms. In the "Case of Sam," he began self-injuring around age eight by burning himself with an eraser, which was not attended to, and his behaviors progressed with age to punching walls and burning. Sam intentionally displayed his injuries to peer groups as a means to garner attention in school. Estimates note that between 8% to 10% of elementary school students as young as in third grade engage in NSSI (Barrocas et al., 2012), and 12% to 25% of secondary school students engage in NSSI (Muehlenkamp et al., 2012; Swannell et al., 2014). A recent study found that 1 in 12 children (8%) engaged in NSSI at least once, and, of that sample, 7.6% were third-graders, 4.0% were sixth graders, and 12.7% were ninthgraders (Barrocas et al., 2012). These findings are alarming and show us that self-injuring is increasing among children. The reason there is an increase in the number of children who self-injure is not clear, but there is a consensus among researchers, mental health providers, and professionals that self-injury is spreading, and some are viewing it as social contagion among youth. Family, internet, media, and peer culture are the vectors that are believed to be increasing the social contagion of NSSI. Additionally, as self-injury in children is now recognized more often, and the diverse nature of clients engaging in self-injury is more readily acknowledged, research is no longer only examining clinical samples, and schools are beginning to become more involved in the mental health concerns of children and reporting the behavior.

Children with intellectual and developmental disabilities (IDDs) are at higher risk for engaging in NSSI (McClintock et al., 2003). Additional risk factors for children can include autism spectrum disorder (ASD), sensory or physical disabilities (Murphy et al., 2005), expression or language difficulties (Richards et al., 2016), and certain genetic disorders (Schroeder et al., 2014). Fodstad et al. (2012) found that in a sample of young children with an IDD (around 10–12 months), 18.3% were engaging in mild forms of self-injurious behaviors (SIB) (eye-poking, self-hitting, and headbanging). Other researchers have found similar SIB within those under five years of age with an IDD (Dimian et al., 2017; Schroeder et al., 2014). Even though these behaviors classify as NSSI, it is crucial to consider that many children with IDDs and ASD can overcome these self-injuring behaviors once they learn to self-soothe, regulate emotions, and engage in verbal expression (if possible). The cognitive and developmental processing of self-injury in younger children is absent or limited, which means they may not clearly understand their behaviors or associated consequences. The pain of the self-injury shifts the focus of the emotional turmoil to the attention of the physical pain. When working with children who may have IDD, the focus of treatment may not necessarily need to be directly on the NSSI, but instead on how to allow the child to express themselves and have their needs met in ways that are not self destructive.

As you begin to consider the age of the client in relation to NSSI, you will notice that the age of onset varies. Roughly 25% of NSSI clients indicate starting between the ages of 10 and 14; 27% between the ages of 15 and 16; and

38.6% between the ages of 17 and 24 (Whitlock et al., 2006). These are crucial developmental periods in teens and young adults. The transition from junior high to high school followed by high school to college can stir up a teenager's/young adult's world. Identity development shifts with these new stressors, and life can become overwhelming if one does not have good coping skills and supports in place. In the "Cases of Rick, Emma, and Charlotte," their NSSI began or increased in severity around times of developmental transition in their educational settings and after periods of trauma. These transitional periods and traumas were not addressed or dealt with directly, causing an increase or onset of NSSI as a coping mechanism.

Even though NSSI is often viewed as a "teen issue or young adult issue," this is not reality. NSSI is documented in adults and elderly populations (Parks & Feldman, 2006). Men over 75 years of age are more likely to engage in self-injury due to health and aging issues that come later in life. NSSI engagement in adolescence often continues to be a problem into adulthood, especially for those who received inadequate or no treatment for the issue. In the "Cases of Jimmy and Dean," both clients had a history of NSSI stemming from adolescence, and neither sought help or treatment. Their methods of self-injurious behaviors are similar to those seen in the adolescent and young adult populations. Now in their later years, they are faced with extreme stressors, therefore NSSI is once again taking over as a coping mechanism. A concrete picture of the prevalence of NSSI in aging adults is difficult to determine due to limited research with aging populations and the stigma that surrounds the act of self-injury into adulthood. This stigma is also likely to cause underreporting when examining prevalence rates of NSSI in the general population (Taylor et al., 2011). Jimmy and Dean both display signs that they are concerned about stigma. They both have not sought treatment for their self-injury and have only disclosed to their partners. The prevalence in those over the age of 30 is reported to be around 5% of the population, which is a quarter of that found for those under 30 in the same study. Additionally, in this same study, NSSI was connected with being younger, unmarried, and with a history of mental health treatment (Klonsky, 2011). Adults with histories of trauma and abuse are more likely to utilize NSSI as a coping mechanism. In the "Case of Rhonda," she began NSSI in her adolescent years but stopped in her 20s while she was with an abusive partner. Since leaving her partner, she has begun engaging in NSSI again. The abusive partner was likely serving a purpose in her life and taking over the role that NSSI used to serve to alleviate her intense emotions. Rhonda has never sought help or treatment for her NSSI, but now that she is on her own, the fear about something happening to her or her children has caused her to seek help.

Many adults who engage in NSSI report it as a way to alleviate negative emotions when they have no affect, while some note that NSSI is a type of self-punishment, a way to communicate, a form of sensation-seeking, or a mechanism for self-distraction (Whitlock et al., 2014) These functions of NSSI are similar to those exhibited by adolescents. While suicide is rarely a co-occurring thought in the act of engaging in NSSI, Joiner's interpersonal-psychological theory finds that acquired ability to engage in NSSI over longer periods may be one of the factors that account for suicide in those with ideation. Suicidal ideation can be high in older adults due to health-related issues, the proximity of social support, and hopelessness. In the "Case of Dean," he recently lost his partner, who was the main person he depended on for social support. He is also living with Parkinson's disease. These developmental and age-related factors make it increasingly challenging for someone like Dean, with an NSSI history, to avoid regressing to injuring as a means of coping. It becomes increasingly difficult to gauge the problem of NSSI in elderly and older adults because, for many, the age of onset was before adulthood, or the person reports having tried NSSI in the past, but without prolonged engagement. Additionally, many adults engage in substance use or abuse and have co-occurring diagnoses, which are also used as a means of coping. Older adults are also more unwilling to disclose their intent or motive around the self-harming behaviors, which seems to be present in the "Case of Jimmy." He has a history of alcohol abuse, narcotics use, and intermittently uses NSSI as a means to cope. His most recent self-injury came after an argument with his wife about his alcohol use. Jimmy was angry and did not want to argue with his wife, but alcohol was not an option to cope since that was the root cause of the argument. Instead, Jimmy knowingly laid his hand on a hot stove. A close relationship has been found between self-harm and suicide in older people who present in hospital settings (Murphy et al., 2012). Suicide and self-harm have shared risk factors. In older and elderly adults, self-neglect is also viewed as a form of self-harm in which the intent is self-destructive behavior used to cope and gain control (Wand et al., 2018). Self-neglect is not a method of NSSI that is typically found in younger populations that self-injure. In the "Case of Dean," he is beginning to self-neglect by refusing to take medication, isolating himself from those around him, and not fulfilling his spiritual needs.

Etiology and function of NSSI

As mentioned throughout Chapter 4, some of the predictors and risk factors for NSSI include having a history of childhood abuse, genetics, poor emotional regulation strategies, parental support and communication, exposure to peer NSSI, other mental health issues or diagnoses, and stressful life events (Arbuthnott & Lewis, 2015; Nock, 2010). While children typically engage in less lethal or severe forms of self-harm as compared to adolescents and adults, understanding what contributes to NSSI in children is critical to preventing ongoing NSSI and to mitigate risk for suicidal behaviors due to prolonged engagement. It is perilous to consider all of the risk and protective factors as you work with your clients to fully assess self-harming behaviors. However, examining risk and protective factors is a critical piece of NSSI assessment, as it helps determine the role or function of NSSI in the client's life. When clinicians can understand the role that NSSI plays in the client's life and the function that it serves, treatment can be further refined to help the client replace the NSSI behaviors with healthy and adaptive coping skills.

Identity development

The biggest question that exists in all of the literature surrounding self-harming behaviors is why people engage in them. Although there are a host of reasons and etiology is always a bit different depending on diversity factors that exist for the client, NSSI is regarded as a way of controlling unwanted thoughts and feelings (Nock, 2010). It is typically best understood as a coping mechanism. Identity formation is one lens through which to view NSSI behaviors. Identity formation is a task of adolescence and early adulthood. Erikson (1993) viewed identity formation as the tension between balancing identity synthesis, which fits together all of the components of identity and identity confusion (i.e., the lack of a clear direction and purpose in life). During identity formation, some central developmental tasks and milestones must be achieved. The failure to take charge and inability to meet these developmental tasks (otherwise known as identity crisis) is hypothesized as a central factor in the onset and preservation of NSSI (Breen et al., 2013). This crisis in identity development can be resolved by fixing the crisis and feeling accomplished, gaining a higher sense of self-esteem and control, or by identity confusion, which can lead to an inability to form close relationships, mood disturbances, disobedience, and possibly psychiatric symptoms. Retrospective understanding of lifetime NSSI has been linked to current identity confusion (Claes et al., 2014). Identity issues may not be the full driving force for NSSI but may influence NSSI behaviors early in life because of their association with other developmental factors that cause the engagement in NSSI (Baetens et al., 2011). NSSI has been correlated with identity development challenges, which cause an inability to cope with negative emotions. Over time, this increases the use of NSSI as a means of emotional regulation, putting the person at higher risk for suicide.

The most common emotion connected with NSSI is shame. Shame is a large component involved in self-injurious acts. Shame is a negative and self-conscious emotion that holds a core belief of being unacceptable or not good enough. Those who experience shame also typically believe that others view them negatively, which is called external shame. External shame leads people to hide parts of themselves in order to avoid rejection (Gilbert, 1998). Shame is a critical emotion to consider when assessing NSSI. When those who self-injure think of themselves as bad or deserving of punishment, it has the potential to intensify the self-injury or make the client want to hide the action from those around them. There is increasing support that links shame as a predictor of NSSI (Schoenleber et al., 2014). For shame-prone individuals, relational and identity-related stressors that trigger shame are managed with NSSI. In the "Case of Charlotte," shame surrounding her identity-related stressors (sexual and gender orientations) could be causing her to use NSSI to cope. Charlotte has not been open with her parents about her gender or sexual orientation, causing her to hide parts of herself. Now that she is in a romantic relationship and cannot share this with her family, the fear and hiding are triggering the feeling of shame.

Theoretical frameworks

Other theories provide a developmental, biological, or neurochemical rationale for the behavior. Developmental differences in early childhood (Erikson, 1993; Piaget, 1964) can cause children to process stressful events differently, potentially resulting in poor coping methods based on the developmental stage. Behavioral theory suggests that early, non-threatening behaviors (e.g., eye touching/rubbing) turn into more severe and frequent acts (e.g., eye-gouging) based on responses from those within the child's environment when the behavior occurs (Guess & Carr, 1991). Adolescence is a distinct developmental period where teens face major decisions and life choices. They also begin to transition to adulthood, a period termed "emerging adulthood." The changes that take place in adolescence are not as obvious as the physical milestones that take place during childhood. Teens struggle with identity development, as well as social, sexual, cognitive, moral, and maturity issues. The thwarted identity development process and psychosocial development process during adolescence and early adulthood are noted to contribute to NSSI behaviors. This age is also a common time for the onset of many mental disorders (Kessler et al., 2005), which makes adolescence itself another risk factor for self-harming behaviors. With all of the changes taking place during adolescence, NSSI can become a maladaptive way to handle internal struggles. For some, this coping mechanism is lasting and takes them into adulthood, while others find healthy coping skills to learn how to overcome challenges. In the "Case of Rick," he is handling several identity development issues. He is in his first romantic relationship and trying to balance his own needs and someone else's. He is also faced with a diagnosis of oppositional defiance disorder and attention deficit disorder as he struggles to find his place with peers and at school. He is expected to make mature decisions now that he is in high school, but he is challenged with trying to incorporate his perceptions and values with those of his father and grandmother.

Biology

There are also biological models of NSSI that focus on the role that NSSI plays in the regulation of endogenous opioids. The homeostasis model of NSSI, for example, suggests that people who self-injure may have chronically low levels of endogenous opioids. In the homeostasis model, NSSI is used as a function to restore opioids to normal levels. Essentially, those who engage in NSSI have low levels of endogenous opioids, which can stem from abuse, trauma, neglect, and so on (Sher & Stanley, 2008). Those who engage in NSSI are found to have increased pain tolerance (Claes et al., 2006), which is said to contribute to the need to engage more frequently or in more destructive ways.

Four-function model

The four-function model (FFM) of non-suicidal self-injury (Nock, 2010) seeks to explain why individuals engage in NSSI. It was developed through research with individuals who have developmental disabilities and posits that NSSI is sustained by four distinct processes that are reinforced due to functionality. There are two dichotomous dimensions that each function falls into: negative vs. positive and automatic (intrapersonal) vs. social (i.e., interpersonal). Automatic negative would be reducing emotional stress and pain, whereas automatic positive would be to increase desired emotional states or feelings. Social negative is to decrease or escape from undesirable social situations and interpersonal demands, and social positive is to increase wanted social situations or garner attention and help-seeking behaviors. A combination of vulnerabilities and difficulty in regulating emotional or social states increases the risk of NSSI engagement (Nock, 2010). The FFM model of NSSI does not fully explain causes of NSSI (biological predispositions and environmental influences), but it goes beyond only identifying psychosocial characteristics associated with NSSI (suicidality and depression), which do not explain why individuals choose to engage in NSSI. FFM classifies self-injury by the specific cause and effect relationships that maintain it, thereby clarifying specific reasons individuals perform NSSI, rather than the relationship between characteristics associated with NSSI. FFM also goes beyond only addressing affect regulation by including automatic and social reinforcement, and distal and specific risk factors, within one comprehensive account.

Assessment of NSSI

The most validated intervention studied for adolescents with NSSI has been said to be the "therapeutic assessment" (Ougrin et al., 2011). In a study by Ougrin et al. (2011), 86% of clients who had a therapeutic assessment attended one or more follow-up appointments compared to 51% of control group clients. This finding demonstrates that the assessment of NSSI is even more critical for the client and clinician. When evaluating youth and adults, simply asking about NSSI behaviors is not enough to gather all of the necessary information. There are many formal assessment measures available that can assist in capturing the complete picture. Though formal assessments offer a piece of information given in a specific time frame, they cannot take the place of building a rapport with your client and gathering all of the information necessary to fully gauge the problem and make accurate decisions about diagnoses and treatment. Since many people who self-harm do not need medical intervention, self-harming information typically is reported directly by your client. These are two primary reasons it is critical that NSSI is correctly assessed: a strong rapport is built with your client, and the client feels they are in a safe enough space to share this information with you. When asking clients about self-injury or suspected self-injury, keep the following practices in mind:

- Respond non-judgmentally, immediately, and directly.
- Avoid shock or emotional displays.
- Don't minimize.

- State that you are there to help and that anything you are asking about or questioning is just because you want to help them to the best of your ability.

If you suspect your client is self-injuring, and he or she has not made this explicit, you can do a discreet visual examination to see if any part of the body that is visible in session has fresh cuts, bruises, or other physical injuries. Additionally, look for any unexplained or clustered scars, marks, and frequent bandages. Parents and caregivers will often be the ones to report these visual indicators to you. Other visual signs could be the use of constant wrist bands or tight bands around the wrist or arm, inappropriate dress for the season, unwillingness to take off jackets or to participate in activities like swimming (again, often parent/caregiver reported).

An initial assessment should include open-ended questions about the behavior. One of the first and most important steps when learning about self-injuring behavior is to assess the intent of self-directed violence. Make sure that there is no intent to die or present suicidal ideation. You want to clearly delineate between the two. Someone with a history of suicide attempts or suicidal ideation would be at a much higher risk, as opposed to someone who does not exhibit these factors. Although self-injury is not necessarily a sign of suicidal ideation, it should be considered as you work with the client. According to Joiner's interpersonal-psychological theory of suicide, someone who self-injures and has a past suicidal ideation history is the highest suicide risk due to the three components that contribute to suicide attempts: thwarted belongingness (alienation from others), ability to act (capacity for suicide), and perceived burdensomeness (view that they are a burden on society). Additionally, you could use a formal assessment of suicidal intent or ideation making sure that suicide is not an immediate risk factor. After it is clear that the self-injury is not an attempt to die, be sure to gather more information related to the risk.

Even if suicidal intent is not present, the following questions are critical:

- Were there any preparatory behaviors before you self-injured, where you knew you were going to injure and got yourself ready? If so, what were they?
- Can you help me to understand, to your knowledge, what purpose the self-injury serves for you?
- Where did the self-injury happen and what was going on or what triggered it (time, place, context, and sequence of events)?
- How were you able to stop the self-injuring in the moment? Did you stop on your own or did someone else intervene?
- Help me to best understand how you knew you were through with the self-injurious behavior. What did it feel like when you knew you were done injuring?
- How long does it usually take you to feel better post-injury?
- After you felt better, what feelings arose?
- Have you ever hurt yourself so badly that you needed medical intervention?

You want to find out about the frequency of self-injury because more repeated and frequent self-injury is more closely related to suicidal ideation. Past suicide attempts are an important piece of information because those who self-injure and have a history of suicide attempts may underestimate the lethality or severity of their self-injuries. Substance use and abuse are critical because clients engaged in these practices are also at higher risk for unintentional suicide attempts. Those who exhibit NSSI in addition to other mental health disorders (such as bulimia and depression) are also at higher risk for suicide attempts and other serious risk concerns. The level of impulsivity in the NSSI should be assessed, along with whether the self-injury is ritualistic or episodic. If the self-injury is based on a ritual and is consistently done at the same time or in the same manner, then it would be approached differently than if the self-injury is used as a way to cope during a distinct episode of distress.

Background information

Gathering background information about your client and the relationship with self-injury is important. It is critical to understand the client's perspectives around the self-injury and what factors are contributing. There should be a focus on how the self-harm serves a purpose in the client's life and the way that it is used to cope. The self-injury should not be dismissed as not important or "silly." The space you create needs to be safe for the client, and you need to be calm and ask questions with respectful curiosity. Respectful curiosity would be asking questions that make the client understand that you want to know more if they will allow it. For example, "help me to better understand ...," or, "if you are able, explain to me ...," which can all help the client to feel less scrutinized or judged. While discussing and assessing the NSSI with the client, there should always be a positive focus on resiliency and the use of a strengths-based approach that is empathetic, supportive, understanding, and encouraging.

This strengths-based approach is also critical when assessing children who engage in NSSI. There are currently no finite NSSI assessments that examine children under 10 that will gauge the entire problem. Also, children at this age have different comprehension levels and may not be able to understand questions on a formal assessment or questions that require deep and reflective thought. This is why a clinician needs a strong rapport with the client and the ability to be adaptable. The clinician should ask simple questions that are clear and also remember that a young child will not have the attention span to answer many questions that will help to assess the injury. The clinician will need to take into account the information that the child client reveals, and also the information offered by those who surround the child, such as parents, siblings, teachers, and close friends. At times, if parents consent, there are assessments that can be given to teachers and guardians to help gauge the problem and give the clinician more information. Some of the clients, such as Jenny and Sam, may not be old enough and far enough along in their cognitive development to answer some of these questions.

When working with children, remember to ask questions that are succinct, use appropriate-level language, and are developmentally appropriate. If you are unable to get some of these questions answered through talk-therapy, you could use play therapy techniques to assist in gathering the information. Sandtray and drawing are two activities that assist younger clients in sharing their stories through their own worldview in a cognitively appropriate way.

Integrated assessment approaches

When assessing and evaluating NSSI, it is necessary to use an integrated approach because of the complex nature of self-injury. Craigen et al. (2010) present a two-tier integrated approach to assess for self-injury (see Figure 5.1). The first step includes utilizing a formal assessment for self-injury, or any other assessment for related diagnoses or concerns. This allows you to make sure that the self-injury is not better explained by other diagnoses or a symptom associated with an additional diagnosis. For example, you could complete a suicide, depression, or trauma inventory. The next tier involves all informal assessments that you may want to conduct. These assessments include any subjective or objective information that you want to gather regarding aspects like family history, social support, emotional capacity, and coping strategies.

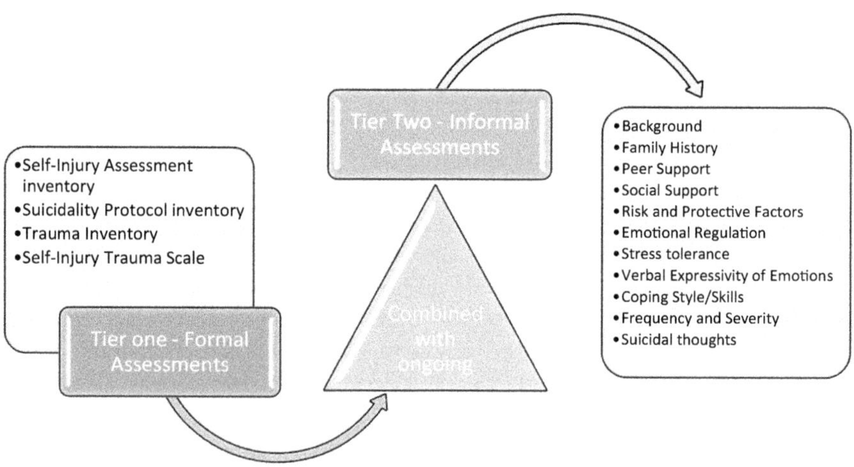

Figure 5.1 Integrated assessment approach.

Stages of change

When assessing NSSI, it is also important to examine the Stage Model of NSSI (Williams et al., 2010) and Prochaska et al. (1992) Model of Readiness for Change. The stage model of NSSI is similar to other models of behavior and allows the clinician to tailor treatment according to the stage. The stages are as follows:

1. Experimental NSSI: the first act of NSSI is attempted, and the client is still determining if they will commit to following through with additional acts of NSSI.
2. Exploration: NSSI is explored via various methods to determine their own physical and psychological responses to the act. Peer or online communities that support the act may be explored and connected to for identification.
3. Encapsulation: NSSI has become the primary coping strategy used to gain emotional control, and the behavior becomes more difficult to hide.
4. Pervasive Dysfunction: the NSSI is not able to be controlled and is the exclusive method used for emotional regulation. The self-injury takes places whenever necessary, and the probability of suicidal thoughts becomes higher as self-injury becomes more frequent and intense.

The Model of Readiness for Change (Figure 5.2) examines the stage of change that the client is currently in. The stages of the model are pre-contemplation, contemplation, preparation, action, and maintenance. When both models are used simultaneously, they have an inverse relationship. As the readiness for change decreases, the stage of NSSI increases.

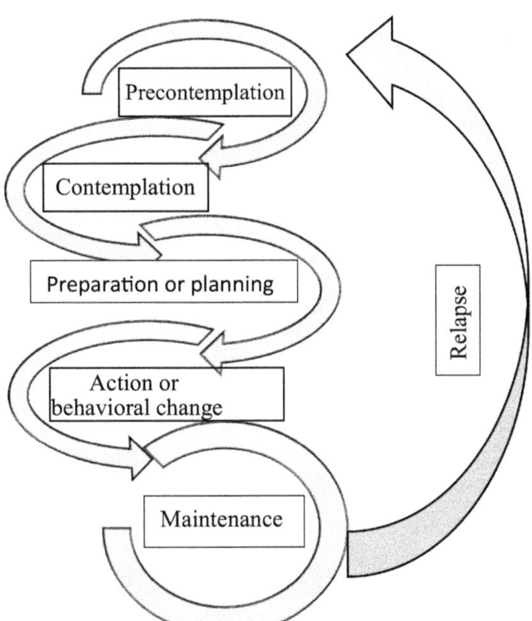

Figure 5.2 Readiness for change stage model.

HIRE model

The HIRE model is another tool for conducting an informal assessment of NSSI. The model is essentially a mnemonic device or acronym to help the clinician remember to assess for each of the domains. This is a great resource for clinicians who may not have experience with NSSI or are new to the field. It assists in gathering information based on diagnostic criteria while keeping safety in mind. The acronym is as follows: H = History, I = Interest in Change, R = Reasons behind Behavior, and E = Exposure to Risk (Buser & Buser, 2013).

STOP FIRE model

The STOP FIRE method is another example of a mnemonic device to help in the assessment of self-injury. It assesses each of the imminent areas of self-injury, so the clinician has all of the pieces of information to make an accurate assessment. The acronym is as follows: S = Suicidal ideations during or before self-injury, T = Types of self-injury in which the patient engages, O = Onset of self-injury, P = Place (location) on the body that is injured, S = Severity and extent of damage caused by self-injury, F = Functions of the self-injury for the patient, I = Intensity or frequency of self-injury urges, R = Repetition of self-injury, and E = Episodic frequency of self-injury. Below you will find dialogue using the STOP FIRE method in the case of Jimmy.

STOP FIRE used with the case of Jimmy

Therapist: Jimmy, I know suicide is very different than self-injuring, but it is important to talk about. Have you ever thought about killing yourself or suicide before, during, or after you engage in self-injury?

Jimmy: In the past, I have, though I have not had suicidal thoughts in a long time.

Therapist: Jimmy, when you are unable to self-injure in order to help you calm down, have you ever had thoughts of suicide? I know you said you have not recently had suicidal thoughts, but I just want to make sure there hasn't been a time more recently.

Jimmy: No, you are correct. The last time was probably about 15 or more years ago.

Therapist: What methods have you used to self-injure currently and in the past?

Jimmy: I have burned myself recently and punched walls and door until I bleed. In the past, I have done similar things and cut myself. My last suicide attempt, which was in my 20s, was an intentional overdose of narcotics. I took the narcotics after I cut myself several times, and nothing was helping me feel better.

Therapist: It sounds like you were really overwhelmed at that moment when the self-injury wasn't working. What happened after you took the narcotics?

Jimmy: A friend at the time found me, and I was in and out of consciousness. They made me vomit, and I finally started to come to.

Therapist: How long have you struggled with suicidal thoughts and self-injury.

Jimmy: My NSSI has been as early as I can remember. My suicidal thoughts began in my early 20s, if not a bit sooner. It is hard to remember.

Therapist: Thanks for all of this information. I know at times it can be challenging to recall, especially since this has been a struggle for some time now. Are there any specific parts of your body that you usually injure? What parts have you injured in the past?

Jimmy: Usually, my hands and arms. I will typically hit with my fists and arms or burn myself with the stove. These are usually areas that I can make excuses for the injuries. Sometimes I hit my hands with objects.

Therapist: Have your injuries ever been severe enough to be hospitalized? If not, how have you addressed your wounds?

Jimmy: Yes, the burns have been bad, and I have taken myself to the hospital, or sometimes my wife has forced me to go. I usually do not like to go to the hospital because of my issues with substance use. I get tempted too easily, and I know I have no self-control. Like once I intentionally missed a nail while hammering and hit my hand. It was very painful, but I refused the pain meds from the hospital.

Therapist: I can imagine that would be very difficult, but you seem to know that drugs and alcohol are a trigger and an area of weakness for you.

Jimmy: Yes, definitely.

Therapist: It sounds like your wife is supportive and tries to assist you when you do self-injure. Do you know why you self-injure? What purpose or function does it serve?

Jimmy: I don't know. I think it is just when I am upset and overwhelmed. I don't know what to do when things go wrong in my relationships, and I am usually to blame. I am so stupid about something, and I don't know how to handle conflict with people. When I am angry at myself, and I can't get the right words out or know I am going to snap; I tend to hurt myself first because it stops me from taking out my impulses in other ways.

Therapist: How do you feel pre- and post- injury?

Jimmy: I am usually worked up and angry toward myself before I injure. Cutting makes me feel relief, but it is usually followed by more guilt because I know my wife will find out and be disappointed.

Therapist: On a scale of 1 to 10 (with 10 being the strongest), how high are your urges to injure every day?

Jimmy: It is not an everyday thing. It is usually about once a week or every two weeks—mainly after arguments with loved ones. I usually don't sweat the small stuff and can fix it. But when people are mad at me, I have no control and cannot find any way to change it. I would say when I am going to injure, the urge is a 10, but most days it is 0.

Therapist: How many times do you think you have self-injured since you started back up again?

Jimmy: That's hard to say. I have injured myself for what feels like forever. Sometimes I can stop for a while, but this past year, I started back up again after my drinking took a turn for the worse. I would say I have self-injured 15 major times this year, with about 10 smaller instances of minor cuts or punches.

Therapist: So, in a typical day, would it be accurate to say you do not self-injure to get through the day?

Jimmy: That is right. It's just when I really don't know what to do with my anger or inability to communicate with those I care for. They usually get onto me about my drinking or say that I should go to a recovery program. Then, I don't know what to do. I become so angry.

Therapist: This was a lot of very helpful information, Jimmy. Thanks for being so open with me. I know it can be hard opening up to someone you don't know and especially about a topic that could be private to you. You did a great job communicating with me today, and I hope we can continue to discuss this in the coming weeks. This information will really help guide me to figure out how to best work together and find a way that will assist you to stop self-injuring.

SOARS model

The SOARS model (Westers et al., 2016) is a brief assessment tool to help clinicians screen for self-harming behavior. It is intended for use by physicians because most often, NSSI will be noticed in a physician's office as opposed to a client reporting the NSSI. The first step when noticing an injury that looks like it could be NSSI will be to ask the client about the injury. Then ask the client if they have ever hurt themselves on purpose without intending to die and to give clear examples. If the client responds affirmatively, you will go through the following model:

1. Suicidal ideation = Check for suicidal ideation. Affirm that you understand that self-injury is not about suicide, but you know that some people may feel that it is about suicide. Then, once you have expressed your understanding, ask directly, "When you injure yourself, do you ever think about purposely ending your life?"
2. Onset, frequency, and methods = Verify the onset of the behavior. "When was the first time and last time you self-injured? How long would you say you have been self-injuring? How often do you self-injure in a day, week, or month? What do you typically use to self-injure, and do you injure in more than one way?"
3. Aftercare = Confirm aftercare practices. "How do you care for yourself and your wound once you are done? Have you ever needed medical attention or someone to stop you from self-injuring further?"
4. Reasons = Clarify the reasons for the behavior. "It sounds like it helps you, and you have a reason for injuring. Would you help me to understand what some of those reasons might be?"
5. Stage of change = Assess if the client is ready for a change. "Is this something you want to stop, or have you ever tried to stop?"

Chain analysis

Chain analysis is a detailed form of assessment that will capture any behavior. It is usually an effective assessment technique to use with kids or teens who may not be able to verbally express themselves or clients who cannot explain what factors caused or led up to their NSSI. The chain will assist clients in making sense of NSSI and orient them to the fact that even though they cannot pinpoint why the NSSI happened, there is a reason. Once they can do this, the client should feel somewhat in control. Initially, you will begin by asking the client to detail the events internally and externally that led up to the most recent incident of self-injury that is clearly remembered. As the client shares the story, you will visually map the details on paper, so they can "see" their story. It may sometimes even help to tell the client that you want as much detail as possible, so you can clearly "write their story or portray the movie." The events, thoughts, emotions, and feelings around the behavior should be detailed. Ask questions about how they got to that place and what specifically pushed them toward the moment when they injured (e.g., if the injury was a cut, you could ask: "What was the moment like right before you began to search for the razor, and while you were searching for it?"). The questions below provide examples of chain analysis:

Thoughts: What were you thinking? What went through your head? Is there anything you said to yourself in your head or out loud?

Feelings: How were you feeling? What kind of mood were you in at the time? What was going on within your body? What was your physical feeling at that moment?

Behaviors: Why did you do it? How did you act? What actions did you take before you injured? When did you know you were going to injure? After you injured?

Vulnerabilities: Why then? Consider sleep, eating, and prior events. What was going on for you? Were other people involved?

Consequences: What happened afterward? Consider reinforcement and punishment. Did you feel better or worse? What did you do with the injury? Did you need medical attention? Did others see it? If so, how did you feel when someone noticed the injury?

Go through the chain with the client and be sure to examine each moment. The client may struggle, but you should reassure him or her that this is okay. Highlight patterns that exist for the client and emphasize anything specific that is important for the client to acknowledge. Identify parts of the chain for the client, such as the point of no return, how to break links between the prompting event and point of no return, and ways to break links between the behavior and consequence. Be sure to review the chain fully with the client, addressing the needs to be fulfilled, feelings after the chain was identified, and how one can respect feelings without giving in emotionally. It is important to validate the client's needs, understand their process, and explore alternatives. A visual representation of a chain analysis activity chart is located in Appendix G.

Formal assessments

Clinicians need to have an understanding of the functions of self-injury before choosing a formal assessment. NSSI is often confused with suicidal behaviors, but they are not the same. This is an issue that needs to be clarified before beginning work with a client. If the intent of the injury is not clear, then a suicide assessment or an NSSI instrument that also examines suicide (such as the Direct and Indirect Self-Harm Inventory) would be useful. Many research tools are available that assess NSSI. The problems are that they often have a limited scope of measurement or have not been rigorously tested to deem their efficacy fully.

Additionally, some scales exist within suicide assessments or fail to fully rule out NSSI with a suicide attempt. As discussed, suicide attempts have fundamental differences from NSSI. When selecting an assessment tool, it is critical that clinicians understand the assessment tool itself and how to administer, score, and interpret results. Clinicians should understand the phenomenon of self-injury and how it continues to evolve. Table 5.2 contains available NSSI assessment tools and the domains they cover. It is important to know the population or person you are assessing and what you specifically want to assess before choosing an assessment tool. Assessments are also only a part of the puzzle in understanding what is going on with the client, which is why integrated approaches, as mentioned above, are critical.

Of the assessments listed above, the Self Injury Trauma Scale (SITS) is one of the most widely used. It was created to evaluate the extent of tissue damage caused by self-injurious behavior and quantifies the tissue damage (Iwata et al., 1990). The Self-Injury Questionnaire (SIQ) was developed to evaluate differentiation in self-injury intentions based on a history of childhood physical and/or sexual abuse, and it defines self-injury as self-destructive behavior without the intent to die (Alexander, 1999). The Self-Injurious Thoughts and Behaviors Interview (SITBI) consists of a 169-item, structured interview to examine the presence, frequency, severity, age of onset, and general characteristics associated with the thoughts and behaviors of suicidal ideations and suicide attempts. This assessment clearly defines self-injury, and it clarifies that self-injury does not include the intent to die; thus, self-injury is differentiated from suicidal intent and action (Nock et al., 2007). The Deliberate Self-Harm Inventory (DSHI) was developed using an integrated definition of self-injury to help provide a clear foundation for the instrument, given that previous assessments had lacked consensus in the definition (Gratz, 2001). It contains 17 items that are behaviorally based and reliant on self-report. The instrument has high internal consistency; adequate construct, convergent, and discriminant validity; and adequate test-retest reliability. Appropriate selection of instruments, along with a critical interview about the self-harming behaviors, will assist counselors in

Table 5.2 Assessments available for NSSI

Assessment name/authors	*Domains measured*	*Availability*	*Psychometric properties*	*Items/format*
Alexian Brothers Assessment of Self Injury Scale (ABASI) Washburn, Potthoff, Juzwin, & Styer	NSSI frequency, methods, functions, DSM-5 criteria, and other characteristics	Available online https://itriples.org/category/measures/	3D, 3E, 2J, 3K	1 & 4 44 items Short form available
Alexian Brothers Urge to Self-Injure Scale (ABUSI) Washburn, Juzwin, Styer, & Aldridge	Past week urges to engage in NSSI	Available online See itriples measures website	3G, 4J, 4K	1 Five items
Attitudes towards Deliberate Self-Harm Questionnaire (ADSHQ) McAllister, Creedy, Moyle, & Farrugia	Attitudes toward NSSI	Available online See itriples measures website	Reliability demonstrated, not specified	1 33 items
Brief Severity Index for Nonsuicidal Self-Injury (BSI-NSSI) Buser, Peterson, & Hill	Identify and distinguish among graduations of NSSI severity	Assessment attached to following article: (2016). Brief Severity Index for Nonsuicidal Self-Injury: Initial validation of a self-report measure. *Journal of Mental Health Counseling*, 38(1), 28–46.	B, L	1 35 items
Brief Non-Suicidal Self Injury-Assessment Tool (BNSSI-AT) Whitlock & Purington	Assess primary and secondary NSSI characteristics	Available online http://www.selfinjury.bctr.cornell.edu/perch/resources/bnssi-at-revised-final-3-3.pdf	B, E, F, J	1, 2, & 3 12 items

(*Continued*)

Table 5.2 (Continued) Assessments available for NSSI

Assessment name/authors	*Domains measured*	*Availability*	*Psychometric properties*	*Items/format*
Clinician-Administered Nonsuicidal Self-Injury Disorder Index (CANDI) Gratz, Dixon-Gordon, Chapman, & Tull	Frequency, severity, duration, and type of NSSI behavior	Email author	3I, 2K	Self-report screening and semi-structured interview
Direct and Indirect Self-Harm Inventory (DISH) Green, Hatgis, Kearns, Nock, & Marx	High-risk behavior, indirect self-harm, NSSI in the past year, reasons/contextual factors, suicidal intent	Email author	3E	20 items
Deliberate Self Harm Inventory (DSHI) Gratz	Developed using an integrated definition of self-injury to help provide a clear foundation for the instrument, as previous assessments had lacked consensus in definition	Email author or see article online http://www.selfinjury.bctr.cornell.edu/perch/resources/deliberate-self-harm-inventory.pdf	2E, 3J, 3K	17 items
Inventory of Statements About Self-Injury (ISAS) Klonsky	NSSI frequency, methods, and functions	Available online http://www2.psych.ubc.ca/~klonsky/publications/ISASmeasure.pdf	4K	1, 2, 3, 4 46 items

(Continued)

Table 5.2 (Continued) Assessments available for NSSI

Assessment name/authors	*Domains measured*	*Availability*	*Psychometric properties*	*Items/format*
NSSI Disorder Scale (NSSIDS) Victor, Davis, & Klonsky	DSM-5 proposed diagnostic criteria for NSSI Disorder	Available online http://www2.psych.ubc.ca/~klonsky/publications/NSSIDS_measure.pdf	3H, 3K	1, 2, 3, 4 16 items
NSSI Expectancy Questionnaire Hasking & Boyes	Expectancies of NSSI (affect regulation, negative social outcomes, communication, pain, negative self-beliefs)	Available online See itriples measures website	4K	1 25 items
NSSI Implicit Association Test (NSSI-IAT) Nock & Banaji	Implicit self-associations with NSSI stimuli	Available online https://www.millisecond.com/download/library/iat/	3D	Computer-based stimuli response
NSSI Scar Cognition Scale (NSSI-SCS) Burke, Olino, & Alloy	NSSI scar cognitions	Available online See itriples measures website	C, E, L	1 26 items
Self-Harm Inventory (SHI) Sansone, Sansone, & Wiederman	Identifies self-injury in conjunction with BPD	Available online See itriples measures website	4D	4 22 items
Self-Injury Motivations Scale (SIMS) Osuch	Self-reported motivation for NSSI	Available online See itriples measures website	4A, 3C, 3D	1 36 items

(*Continued*)

Table 5.2 (Continued) Assessments available for NSSI

Assessment name/authors	*Domains measured*	*Availability*	*Psychometric properties*	*Items/format*
Self-Injury Trauma Scale (SITS) Iwata, Pace, & Kissel	Predict current risk	Assessment attached to the following article: (1990). The Self-Injury Trauma (SIT) scale: A method for quantifying surface tissue damage caused by self-injurious behavior. *Journal of Applied Behavior Analysis*, 23(2), 99–110.	3J, 4K	2 & 3
Self-Injury Questionnaire (SIQ) Alexander	Intentions for self-harm per method across four subscales	Available online https://itriples.org/wp-content/uploads/measures/Web_SIQ.pdf	4H, 4K	1, 2, 3, & 4 30 items
Self-Injury Questionnaire – Treatment Related (SIQ-TR) Claes & Vandereycken	Type, frequency, duration, and functions of NSSI, affective antecedents and consequences	Available online See itriples measures website	K, M	1 & 2 60 items
Structured Interview for Self-Destructive Behavior (SI-SDB) Carlson, Armstrong & Loewenstein	Frequency, age of onset, scarring, and methods of NSSI, assessment of suicidality, risky sexual behavior, substance use, and disordered eating	Available online See itriples measures website		1 & 5 5 items

(*Continued*)

Table 5.2 (Continued) Assessments available for NSSI

Assessment name/authors	*Domains measured*	*Availability*	*Psychometric properties*	*Items/format*
Self-Injurious Thoughts and Behaviors Interview (SITBI) Nock, Holmberg, Photos, & Michel	To assess a wide range of self-injury-related constructs	Available online https://itriples.org/category/measures/	2H, 4I, 3J	5 169 items Short form available
Functional Assessment of Self-Mutilation Lloyd, Kelley, & Hope	Assess the methods, frequency and functions of self-reported NSSI	Available online See itriples measures website	2C, 2K	1 & 3
Suicide Attempt Self-Injury Interview (SASII) Linehan, Comtois, Brown, Heard, & Wagner	Assesses the factors involved in non-fatal suicide attempts and intentional self-injury	Available online http://depts.washington.edu/uwbrtc/resources/assessment-instruments/	4I, 3M	1, 3, & 4

Psychometric properties codes:

1 = poor, 2 = moderate, 3 = good, 4 = excellent

A = face validity, B = content validity, C = concurrent validity, D = predictive validity, E = convergent validity, F = discriminant validity, G = incremental validity, H = construct validity, I = inter-rater reliability, J = test-retest reliability, K = internal consistency reliability, L = reliability not specified, M = validity not specified

Items/format codes:

1 = Likert scale, 2 = multiple choice, 3 = open-ended, 4 = closed-ended, 5 = structured interview.

Age/gender codes:

1 = children, 2 = adolescents, 3 = adults, 4 = older adults; A = female, B = male

putting the pieces of the puzzle together. A single assessment, used in isolation, is only part of the puzzle for that moment in time. It should never be used in isolation. Appropriate assessment selection and interviews will help guide treatment focus and assist you in making a comprehensive treatment plan. There are many steps involved, so, if needed, use a checklist that will help keep you on track and ensure that you have thoroughly evaluated and assessed your client (see Appendix H for a sample checklist).

REFERENCES

Alexander, L. (1999). *The functions of self-injury and its link to traumatic events in college students* (Doctoral dissertation). Retrieved from *UMI Dissertation Services*. (UMI No. 9932285)

American Psychiatric Association. (2013). *Diagnostic and Statistical Manual of Mental Disorders (DSM-5)*. Washington, DC: American Psychiatric Association Publishing.

Arbuthnott, A.E., & Lewis, S.P. (2015). Parents of youth who self-injure: A review of the literature and implications for mental health professionals. *Child and Adolescent Psychiatry and Mental Health*, 9(1), 35. doi:10.1186/s13034-015-0066-3

Baetens, I., Claes, L., Willem, L., Muehlenkamp, J., & Bijttebier, P. (2011). The relationship between non-suicidal self-injury and temperament in male and female adolescents based on child-and parent-report. *Personality and Individual Differences*, 50(4), 527–530. doi:10.1016/j.paid.2010.11.015

Barrocas, A.L., Hankin, B.L., Young, J.F., & Abela, J.R. (2012). Rates of nonsuicidal self-injury in youth: Age, sex, and behavioral methods in a community sample. *Pediatrics*, 130(1), 39–45. doi:10.1542/peds.2011-2094

Breen, A.V., Lewis, S.P., & Sutherland, O. (2013). Brief report: Non-suicidal self-injury in the context of self and identity development. *Journal of Adult Development*, 20, 57–62. doi:10.1007/s10804-013-9156-8

Buser, T., & Buser, J. (2013). The HIRE model: A tool for the informal assessment of nonsuicidal self-injury. *Journal of Mental Health Counseling*, 35(3), 262–281. doi:10.17744/mehc.35.3.h27684682833phk1

Centers for Disease Control and Prevention. (2014). National Suicide Statistics. Retrieved from https://www.cdc.gov/violenceprevention/suicide/statistics.html

Claes, L., Luyckx, K., & Bijttebier, P. (2014). Non-suicidal self-injury in adolescents: Prevalence and associations with identity formation above and beyond depression. *Personality and Individual Differences*, 61, 101–104.

Claes, L., Vandereycken, W., & Vertommen, H. (2006). Pain experience related to self-injury in eating disorder patients. *Eating behaviors*, 7(3), 204–213. doi:10.1016/j.eatbeh.2005.09.003

Craigen, L.M., Healey, A.C., Walley, C.T., Byrd, R., & Schuster, J. (2010). Assessment and self-injury: Implications for counselors. *Measurement and Evaluation in Counseling and Development*, 43(1), 3–15. doi:10.1177/0748175610362237

Dimian, A.F., Botteron, K.N., Dager, S.R., Elison, J.T., Estes, A.M., Pruett, J.R., … Wolff, J. (2017). Potential risk factors for the development of self-injurious behavior among infants at risk for Autism Spectrum Disorder. *Journal of Autism and Developmental Disorders*, 47(5), 1403–1415. doi:10.1007/s10803-017-3057-9

Erikson, E.H. (1993). *Childhood and Society*. New York, NY: WW Norton & Company.

Fodstad, J.C., Rojahn, J., & Matson, J.L. (2012). The emergence of challenging behaviors in at-risk toddlers with and without autism spectrum disorder: A cross-sectional study. *Journal of Developmental and Physical Disabilities*, 24(3), 217–234. doi:10.1007/s10882-011-9266-9

Gilbert, P. (1998). What is shame? Some core issues and controversies. In: P. Gilbert & B. Andrews (Eds.), *Shame: Interpersonal Behavior, Psychopathology*. Oxford, UK: Oxford University Press.

Gratz, K.L. (2001). Measurement of deliberate self-harm: Preliminary data on the deliberate self-harm inventory. *Journal of Psychopathology and Behavioral Assessment*, 23(4), 253–263.

Guess, D., & Carr, E. (1991). Emergence and maintenance of stereotypy and self-injury. *American Journal on Mental Retardation*, 96(3), 299–319

Iwata, B.A., Pace, G.M., Kissel, R.C., Nau, P.A., & Farber, J.M. (1990). The self-injury trauma (SIT) scale: A method for quantifying surface tissue damage caused by self-injurious behavior. *Journal of Applied Behavior Analysis*, 23(1), 99–110. doi:10.1901/jaba.1990.23-99

Joiner, T. (2007). *Why People Die by Suicide*. Cambridge, MA: Harvard University Press.

Kessler, R.C., Berglund, P., Demler, O., Jin, R., Merikangas, K.R., & Walters, E.E. (2005). Lifetime prevalence and age-of-onset distributions of DSM-IV disorders in the National Comorbidity Survey Replication. *Archives of general psychiatry*, 62(6), 593–602. doi:10.1001/archpsyc.62.6.593

Klonsky, E.D. (2011). Non-suicidal self-injury in United States adults: Prevalence, sociodemographics, topography and functions. *Psychological Medicine*, 41(9), 1981–1986. doi:10.1017/s0033291710002497

Lofthouse, N.L., Muehlenkamp, J.J., & Adler, R. (2008). Nonsuicidal self-injury and co-occurrence. In M.K. Nixon & N.L. Heath (Eds.), *Self-Injury in Youth: The Essential Guide to Assessment and Intervention* (pp. 59–78). New York, NY: Routledge. doi:10.4324/9780203892671

Madge, N., Hewitt, A., Hawton, K., de Wilde, E.J., Corcoran, P., Fekete S., … Ystgaard, M. (2008). Deliberate self-harm within an international community sample of young people: Comparative findings from the Child and Adolescent Self-Harm in Europe (CASE) Study. *Journal of Child Psychology and Psychiatry*, 49, 667–677. doi:10.1111/j.1469-7610.2008.01879.x

McClintock, K., Hall, S., & Oliver, C. (2003). Risk markers associated with challenging behaviours in people with intellectual disabilities: A meta-analytic study. *Journal of Intellectual Disability Research*, 47(6), 405–416. doi:10.1046/j.1365-2788.2003.00517.x

Muehlenkamp, J.J., Claes, L., Havertape, L., & Plener, P.L. (2012). International prevalence of adolescent non-suicidal self-injury and deliberate self-harm. *Child and Adolescent Psychiatry and Mental Health*, 6(1), 10. doi:10.1186/1753-2000-6-10

Murphy, E., Kapur, N., Webb, R., Purandare, N., Hawton, K., Bergen, H., … Cooper, J. (2012). Risk factors for repetition and suicide following selfharm in older adults: Multicentre cohort study. *British Journal of Psychiatry*, 200(5), 399–404. doi:10.1192/bjp.bp.111.094177

Murphy, G.H., Beadle-Brown, J., Wing, L., Gould, J., Shah, A., & Holmes, N. (2005). Chronicity of challenging behaviours in people with severe intellectual disabilities and/or autism: A total population sample. *Journal of Autism and Developmental Disorders*, 35(4), 405–418. doi:10.1007/s10803-005-5030-2

Nock, M.K. (2010). Self-injury. *Annual Review of Clinical Psychology*, 6, 339–363. doi:10.1146/annurev.clinpsy.121208.131258

Nock, M.K., Holmberg, E.B., Photos, V.I., & Michel, B.D. (2007). Self-injurious thoughts and behaviors interview: Development, reliability and validity in an adolescent sample. *Psychological Assessment*, 19(3), 309–317. doi:10.1037/1040-3590.19.3.309

Nock, M.K., Joiner, T.E. Jr., Gordon, K.H., Lloyd-Richardson, E., & Prinstein, M.J. (2006). Nonsuicidal self-injury among adolescents: Diagnostic correlates and relation to suicide attempts. *Psychiatry Research*, 144(1), 65–72. doi:10.1016/j.psychres.2006.05.010

Ougrin, D., Zundel, T., Ng, A., Banarsee, R., Bottle, A., & Taylor, E. (2011). Trial of therapeutic assessment in London: Randomised controlled trial of therapeutic assessment versus standard psychosocial assessment in adolescents presenting with self-harm. *Archives of Disease in Childhood*, 96, 148–153. doi:10.1136/adc.2010.188755

Parks, S.M., & Feldman, S.M. (2006). Self-injurious behavior in the elderly. *The Consultant Pharmacist: The Journal of the American Society of Consultant Pharmacists*, 21, 905–910. doi:10.4140/tcp.n.2006.905

Piaget, J. (1964). Part I: Cognitive development in children: Piaget development and learning. *Journal of Research in Science Teaching*, 2(3), 176–186. doi:10.1002/tea.3660020306

Prochaska, J.O., DiClemente, C.C., & Norcross, J.C. (1992). In search of how people change: Applications to addictive behaviors. *American Psychologist*, 47(9), 1102. doi:10.1037//0003-066x.47.9.1102

Richards, C., Moss, J., Nelson, L., & Oliver, C. (2016). Persistence of self-injurious behaviour in autism spectrum disorder over 3 years: A prospective cohort study of risk markers. *Journal of Neurodevelopmental Disorders*, 8(1), 21. doi:10.1186/s11689-016-9153-x

Rowe, S.L., French, R.S., Henderson, C., Ougrin, D., Slade, M., & Moran, P. (2014). Help-seeking behaviour and adolescent self-harm: A systematic review. *Australian & New Zealand Journal of Psychiatry*, 48(12), 1083–1095. doi:10.1177/0004867414555718

Schoenleber, M., Berenbaum, H., & Motl, R. (2014). Shame-related functions of and motivations for self-injurious behavior. *Personality Disorders: Theory, Research, & Treatment*, 5, 204–211. doi:10.1037/per0000035

Schroeder, S.R., Marquis, J.G., Reese, R.M., Richman, D.M., Mayo-Ortega, L., Oyama-Ganiko, R., … Lawrence, L. (2014). Risk factors for self-injury, aggression, and stereotyped behavior among young children at risk for intellectual and developmental disabilities. *American Journal on Intellectual and Developmental Disabilities*, 119(4), 351–370. doi:10.1352/1944-7558-119.4.351

Sher, L., & Stanley, B.H. (2008). The role of endogenous opioids in the pathophysiology of self-injurious and suicidal behavior. *Archives of Suicide Research*, 12(4), 299–308. doi:10.1080/13811110802324748

Swannell, S.V., Martin, G.E., Page, A., Hasking, P., & St John, N.J. (2014). Prevalence of nonsuicidal self-injury in nonclinical samples: Systematic review, meta-analysis and meta-regression. *Suicide and Life-Threatening Behavior*, 44(3), 273–303. doi:10.1111/sltb.12070

Taylor, A.W., Martin, G., Dal Grande, E., Swannell, S., Fullerton, S., Hazell, P., & Harrison, J.E. (2011). Methodological issues associated with collecting sensitive information over the telephone—Experience from an Australian non-suicidal self-injury (NSSI) prevalence study. *BMC Medical Research Methodology*, 11(1), 20. doi:10.1186/1471-2288-11-20

Wand, A.P.F., Peisah, C., Draper, B., & Brodaty, H. (2018). Understanding self-harm in older people: A systematic review of qualitative studies. *Aging & Mental Health*, 22(3), 289–298. doi:10.1080/13607863.2017.1304522

Westers, N.J., Muehlenkamp, J.J., & Lau, M. (2016). SOARS model: Risk assessment of nonsuicidal self-injury. *Contemporary Pediatrics*, 33(7), 25–31.

Whitlock, J., Eckenrode, J., & Silverman, D. (2006). Self-injurious behaviors in a college population. *Pediatrics*, 117(6), 1939–1948. doi:10.1542/peds.2005-2543

Whitlock, J., Exner-Cortens, D., & Purington, A. (2014). Assessment of nonsuicidal self-injury: Development and initial validation of the Non-Suicidal Self-Injury Assessment Tool (NSSI-AT). *Psychological Assessment*, 26(3), 935. doi:10.1037/a0036611

Williams, E., Daley, A., & Iennaco, J. (2010). Assessing non-suicidal self-injurious behaviours in adolescents. *American Journal of Nurse Practitioners*, 14(5), 18–20.

6 Gender and cultural considerations

Kelly Emelianchik-Key

Developmental variations in early childhood (Erikson, 1993; Piaget, 1958) can cause children to process stressful events differently, potentially resulting in poor coping methods based on the developmental stage of the child. Childhood, adolescence, and young adulthood are marked by transitional periods that link to the process of identity development salient to ones' eventual transition into adulthood (Arnett, 2000). These developmental periods can contribute to times of increased confusion depending on environmental factors, such as parental influences, social development, and peer groups. Poor adjustment to any of these stages could result in the development of unhealthy coping patterns. Throughout the developmental stages experienced in the lifespan, gender, racial, and cultural identities are shaped and formed. Conflict associated with these areas of identity can also influence the development and use of NSSI when coping becomes problematic. These typical developmental challenges will influence the ways NSSI manifests as the behavior intersects with culture, gender, and diversity issues specific to the context of an individual's life experience. Identity development includes aspects of gender, race, ethnicity, and sexual orientation and all have been shown to influence the process of self-injury in various ways, some of which include presentation, function, the method of self-injury, help-seeking behaviors, and treatment. Various case scenarios with relevant culture and diversity perspectives are present below to highlight relevant contextual factors that coincide with NSSI in the literature.

Identity development

As discussed in Chapter 1, identity development plays a large role in the interpersonal processes that people undergo within their cultural contexts to find out who they are and where they fit in or belong. Identity development starts in childhood. NSSI is a method that can be used to cope with stressors and mood states during development. However, according to some theories, identity development extends through adulthood (Arnett, 2000), and identity is constantly adapting. Erikson (1968) has noted that a secure and healthy adult identity is composed of past, current, and future events. Self-esteem, self-concept, and depression are threats to identity development in adulthood (Harter, 2012).

People who engage in NSSI are viewed as those with identity development challenges who struggle to integrate past, current, and future events. NSSI reveals the visible connection to the self, and it is viewed as a way for some people to bring together these spans of times to help a person counteract the perceived loss of self in adulthood; thus, for some, it serves as an anti-suicide function (Breen et al., 2013).

In the adolescent population, identity development is positively connected to identity synthesis, optimal functioning, and lowered symptomatology (NSSI). Identity confusion is a risk factor often correlated to increased depression and lower perceived well-being (Kroger & Marcia, 2011). However, there is conflicting information, as other studies have found NSSI to be positively related to depression and identity confusion (Breen et al., 2013). Identity confusion is better explained in the presence/absence of NSSI above and beyond gender, age, and depression. NSSI is often viewed as a consequence or a coping strategy to deal with the struggles of the developing self and identity, but it is possible that the presence of NSSI could cause identity confusion over time (Claes et al., 2014). Identity development encompasses more than just identity of self, but it also includes aspects like physical, cognitive, gender identity, and racial identity development. Each of these areas of development is entangled with the healthy development of self-identity and self-concept. Failure or interruptions in any of these areas can also be a risk factor, consequence, or reason for prolonged NSSI engagement.

Gender development

Gender is likely the most prominent attribute about a person, often assigned at birth. However, gender is a socially and culturally constructed definition of what makes a man and a woman. Sex is what biologically makes someone a male or female. When babies are born, we assign a sex to that child per their biological makeup. Then, from there, they are usually assigned a gender, and gender-related characteristics quickly progress before sexual maturity. Gender awareness emerges very early on in development, and its effects are pervasive. There are many theories of gender role development, but most fall within two categories, biological and social-cognitive.

Biological theories

Biological approaches find no differences between sex and gender, suggest that gender is determined by hormones and chromosomes, and are the basis for the gender role distinctions between males and females. Some biological approaches also consider environmental influences. Money and Ehrhardt's (1972) biosocial theory examines the way social and biological factors play a role in gender development by looking at how early gendered socialization experiences impact prenatal biological developments and hormonal influences. Biological theories explain a great deal regarding biologically related influences on gender role development, but most do not account for social-cognitive influences and impacts.

Cognitive theories

These theories emphasize the ways mental representations and social experiences direct and guide gender role behaviors. One of the most notable is Lawrence Kohlberg's (1966) *Gender Consistency Theory*. Children progress through gender development in three stages. Essentially, children think about the experiences they have with both genders, they self-identify, then an understanding or awareness is gained, and boy or girl behaviors are adopted. A full understanding of gender constancy is needed before children engage in the self-initiated gender socialization processes. Table 6.1 contains the stages in Kohlberg's theory.

Table 6.1 Kohlberg's gender consistency theory

Stage	*Task*
Gender Identity 2–3 years old	Self-label and identify as a boy or girl.
Gender Stability 4–5 years old	An understanding that they are and have been a boy or girl.
Gender Consistency 6–7 years old	The realization that appearances can change, but they will not change gender.

Other theories

Other cognitive developmental theories of gender include Sandra Bem's (1983) gender schema theory and Albert Bandura's (1986) social cognitive theory. Gender schema theory is a variation on Kohlberg's theory, and it notes that a basic understanding of gender identity is enough to start the self-initiated gender socialization process in children. Then, gender schema are formed. These are mental representations of what is male and female. As children develop, they advance gendered schema by deciphering what is male and female and determining acceptable male and female activities for self-engagement (Bem, 1983). Social cognitive theory proposes that a concept of gender is developed from: (a) modeling and observing gender-relevant behaviors, (b) learning that gender is relevant and related to consequences experienced through actions, and (c) receiving directed instruction regarding what is appropriate for boys or girls. Self-efficacy influences the development of gender-related knowledge and skills in children (Bandura, 1986).

Gender role conflict and NSSI

Gender role development can affect all areas of development. An overarching theme in all developmental theories is that conflict in gender role development leads to recurrent stress on cognitive and emotional processes. This stress is often brought about by stigma and societal norms placed on gender development, which causes a negative emotional state labeled gender role conflict (GRC). Depression, anxiety, and isolation are associated with GRC. There are also several groups or populations that have been found to struggle with GRC more often than others (e.g., veterans, various racial groups, and various sexual orientations). GRC and NSSI are highly interrelated. NSSI is thought to be the coping mechanism used to deal with the stress of GRC. Research has shown that GRC statistically predicts NSSI frequency (Schillinger & Andover, 2016) in males. Depression accounts for this relationship.

Men's negative attitudes toward help-seeking have been attributed to increased gender role conflict (O'Neil, 2008; Pederson & Vogel, 2007; Wester et al., 2010). Higher states of GRC have been associated with those who have negative attitudes regarding therapy (Pederson & Vogel, 2007; Wester et al., 2010). Blazina et al. (2007) found that many traditionally socialized men will avoid activities that appear feminine or for women (such as seeking social support) to increase their masculine identity. GRC is thought to cause internal turmoil in men, which affects their ability to receive messages about the potential benefits of therapy. Although this interpretation of men and health behaviors is "static," it coincides with characteristics of males. NSSI is frequently seen as a female issue, which can increase stigma and GRC. This could make it even less likely that males who self-injure will seek help or report self-injuring behaviors for fear of being viewed in a feminine way. Social support can positively affect the connection between restricted emotional expression and negative psychological outcomes (e.g., NSSI). Men's inability to seek social support and restricted emotional expression could be one reason NSSI is often found to be more prevalent in females. Women use NSSI as a means to seek support and get help before the NSSI becomes pervasive. Women also have more suicidal ideation but do not have as many completed suicides as males. Males attempt and complete suicide more often than females, which might be due to GRC. GRC does not allow males to seek help as readily as females. They use NSSI as a means to cope, but do not seek social support and express their emotions, which in turn results in more completed suicides. Finding social support outlets is critical for males and females engaging in NSSI (see Appendix I for a social support circle activity).

GRC has also been noted to explain suicidal behaviors in adolescents (Gough & Robertson, 2010; O'Neil, 2008). There are strong similarities and overlap between NSSI and suicidal behaviors, but with clear differences in the two types of behavior regarding representation of traits and willingness (Klonsky & Muehlenkamp, 2007; Messer & Fremouw, 2008). GRC and suicidal behaviors in adolescent males are within the gender patterns of self-injurious behaviors in an adolescent. Self-injury in males presents itself differently regarding physical injury, mood, psychological traits, and interpersonal interactions (Crowell et al., 2008; Wang, 2010). Violent experiences in males are known to lead to negative moods states, such as anger, depression, and anxiety, and they are representative of the interpersonal interactions and relationships between peers, parents, teachers, and various others in a variety of environments (Tipper, 1997; Welsh et al., 1995), but also strongly represent the negative interpersonal interactions in which adolescents are involved.

Gender differences in NSSI

Gender plays a central role in NSSI manifestation. Research is mixed regarding gender and NSSI engagement, with some studies showing more female youth engagement in NSSI when compared with male youth (Laye-Gindhu & Schonert-Reichl, 2005), and other studies showing no gender differences (Gratz et al., 2012). It is difficult to say that NSSI is a female issue, although it is traditionally assumed. From what is known, adolescence and young adulthood is the time when the number of females who engage in NSSI increases significantly. But when looking at younger youth (i.e., third through sixth graders), Barrocas et al. (2012) found that rates of NSSI did not differ between genders. This information coincides with gender role development. Younger children are still exploring their gender identity and fitting together all of the interpersonal and environmental factors. Gender only begins to play a role beginning in ninth grade, suggesting that the transition to adolescence has a strong impact on the prevalence of NSSI. This transition includes conforming to gender roles and perceptions, stigma, peer relationships, changing between schools, and biological changes in hormones as youth begin puberty.

When examining forms and ways of self-injuring, the gender and developmental stage also play a role. Traditionally, adolescent and young adult females report cutting themselves more often (Gratz et al., 2012). Barrocas et al. (2012) found that girls reported cutting or carving their skin most often, while boys reported more frequent instances of hitting themselves. When examining male youths, ninth-grade boys described cutting/carving their skin most often, whereas third-grade boys noted hitting themselves most often. Many of the youth in this study also reported hair-pulling to inflict pain, biting, running into walls, and throwing their body into sharp objects. From this study alone, it seems vital to consider developmental trends and gender when conceptualizing and assessing NSSI behaviors. Whitlock et al. (2011) maintain that behaviors labeled as traditional male expressions of anger have an NSSI component, which includes punching things, shooting staples into body parts, smashing cans on heads (Nock, 2008), betting/daring friends to self-injure, and picking fights with others. Evidence suggests that these, and similar behaviors, are linked to traditional male norms (Cohn et al., 2010), but determining if these behaviors are forms of NSSI can be extremely difficult. Some of these forms of masculine expressions of anger also coincide with the positive association of being a bully as well as NSSI used as an outlet to help with depressive symptoms and emotional regulation (Claes et al., 2015).

Not all studies have found gender differences in the prevalence rates of NSSI (Claes et al., 2014), but those that report differences find a higher risk for women who engage in NSSI. Compared to findings in male populations, NSSI in women is shown to be connected to frequent and highly stressful events (Plener et al., 2009). There is a large amount of research that shows men and women control emotions differently (Kwon et al., 2013; Nolen-Hoeksema, 2012). One example of this is that women tend to use different ways of thinking to process emotions and typically ruminate longer, which could be a contributing factor to higher rates of depression and anxiety among females. When examining adolescent research, girls experience stronger emotional reactivity to stress when compared to boys (Hankin et al., 2007), which again could contribute to more females engaging in NSSI.

Conversely, males more often regulate emotions through the use of aggression and alcohol (Nolen-Hoeksema, 2012), which could contribute to the higher number of male externalizing disorders, such as substance use disorders and antisocial personality disorder. It could also be a reason males follow through with suicide attempts in more lethal ways (e.g., use of firearms). Men are more likely than women to engage in impulsive and severe self-harming behaviors, which adds another concern for clinicians working with males engaging in NSSI. The methods used can be more severe, requiring medical attention. When taking Nock's interpersonal theory of suicide into consideration, more severe and frequent engagement in NSSI behavior relates to the acquired ability to make a suicide attempt. Various forms of NSSI are more socially acceptable for men to engage in versus women. Men are also more likely to engage in burning and self-hitting, which are direct, intentional, and conscious forms of NSSI (Green & Jakupcak, 2016; Whitlock et al., 2011). Males also tend to injure in groups or to let others injure them, as opposed to women, who typically prefer to injure alone.

Culture and diversity

In addition to gender, cultural contexts and diversity greatly influence suicide and self-harming behaviors (Colucci et al., 2013). In the DSM-5, culture is an important mitigating factor contributing to the meaning and definition of NSSI. Unfortunately, there is not much information concerning various cultural groups and the manifestation of self-injury. Most of the research is steeped in Western cultures (Chesin et al., 2013; Gratz et al., 2012). This can often cause researchers to unintentionally disregard the norms and values of different populations that are not like Western cultures. Race, ethnicity, and culture must be taken into consideration when examining NSSI to understand the phenomenon further. The last part of the definition for NSSI from the International Society for the Study of Self-Injury (ISSSI) notes that, "NSSI behaviors that may cause damage but are acceptable in our society, or part of a recognized cultural, spiritual or religious ritual, are not considered self-injury" (ISSSI, 2019). For some cultural groups, self-harm and self-injury are viewed as a ritual for healing or promoting spirituality. In many Western countries, body modifications, body piercing, or tattooing are not viewed as self-injury because of the cultural acceptance of the practice. This is important to note when assessing and addressing self-injury. Clinicians should not be diagnosing something that is part of someone's cultural norm.

Racial groups

Few studies examine ethnic and racial differences in NSSI onset and engagement, and often those that do have underrepresented samples. This makes it challenging to assess NSSI within diverse groups. Whitlock et al. (2006) found Asian Americans to be less likely than other groups to report self-harming behaviors (but African Americans were underrepresented in the sample), while another study found NSSI was more likely to be reported in adolescents who had identified as Black or Other (mostly Native Americans) (Yates et al., 2008). Mixed races are identified as a higher risk group for NSSI engagement (Gratz, 2006; Kuentzel et al., 2012), whereas other small studies with ethnically diverse samples found no difference by race (Yates et al., 2008).

As you can see, most studies that examined NSSI by race have been inconclusive. NSSI has been noted to function interpersonally and intrapersonally. These interpersonal and intrapersonal functions are likely to have connections with specific populations, diversity factors, and cultural origins, but limited studies make finite connections to NSSI engagement or risk factors. Wester and Trepal (2015) addressed the uniqueness inherent in different cultural groups that could contribute to NSSI engagement. In a sample of college students, African Americans and Asian Americans were found to have a significantly lower engagement in self-injurious behaviors when compared to all other racial groups. Hispanic, Multiracial/Other, and Caucasian students did not differ from each other in rates of engagement in NSSI behaviors (Wester & Trepal, 2015). The researchers examined the concepts of ethnic identity and ethnic belonging and found that when culture was a consideration, ethnic belonging served as a possible protective factor for African Americans and Asian American students in the study. This finding is unique and needs further exploration, especially with multiracial populations. A lack of belonging or weak sense of cultural identity could contribute to higher risk for NSSI prevalence. Inherent cultural values and variables need to be examined to understand further how culture and race play a role in NSSI.

Minority stress

Minority stress arises when there are high levels of stress faced by members of a stigmatized minority group. Social and psychological theoretical orientations describe it as the interplay between minority and dominant values, which results in conflict with the social environment experienced by the minority group members (Meyer, 2003). This causes the minority group to be more vulnerable to psychological stress and emotional dysregulation. Poor social support and low socioeconomic status are connected to high minority stress. The members of the minority group often face more discrimination, which leads to physiological stress, poor physical health, and poor mental health. The topic of minority stress has been largely studied in sexual and racial minorities, and research has examined the ways that discrimination (i.e., homophobia, racism, discrimination, and harassment) has affected mental and physical health (Landrine et al., 2006).

Minority stress displays itself differently in various groups based on personal experiences. Minority stress can arise from actual victimization (like bullying or harassment) and from perceived discrimination (where you feel like you are being discriminated against but cannot prove it). Physical and verbal bullying or harassment from minority status causes substantial suffering in mental health issues that may go unrecognized. NSSI is sometimes an unnoticeable coping mechanism that can be used to deal with minority stress. Sexual minorities experience stress from the following factors: hiding sexual orientation, discrimination, oppression, internalized homophobia, and heteronormativity. Overall, ethnic and sexual minorities (i.e., those who are not white and heterosexual) are susceptible to worse physical and mental health due to stress-related factors that are inherent in all areas (educational environments, work settings, neighborhoods, quality of health care, and access to services).

The cases of Jenny and Sam

Jenny and Sam are our two young people engaged in self-injury. Even though they are both similar in age and at the same stage in cognitive development, their cases of NSSI present very differently. Risk and protective factors, in these cases, vary considerably due to their contexts. They are distinct clients when we consider issues specific to gender and cultural experience in relation to their development.

Jenny is a female of multiple heritage (Asian, African American, and Caucasian). Given the available research on race and non-suicidal self-injury, those of multiple ethnic and racial identities could be at an increased risk for NSSI behaviors due to minority stress and issues related to multiple heritage identity development. If Jenny experiences a lack of belongingness or a weak sense of cultural identity, this could affect the frequency and severity of her NSSI behaviors. We are not sure how Jenny views herself in relation to other children her age. During this stage of development, Jenny is trying to feel a sense of accomplishment or success in her abilities, build a sense of identity, and develop peer relationships. The way she views herself compared to others is critical. Are there other students like her in the classroom? During early childhood, kids do not understand differences in terms of identity and thus often disregard racial and gender differences (unless taught otherwise). As children develop, they start to perceive differences, but they also seek out ways to make sense of these differences. Visual cues are important in helping kids make sense of the world, as visual cues are often one of the first senses children use to acknowledge and appreciate diversity as they get older. If Jenny does not see others who are like her, this could affect how she views herself. She may feel alone or that she needs to find other ways of fitting in, which could give her a greater sense of urgency to be "perfect" as she sees it defined by others. Jenny is receiving support from her teachers and those around her. This could be because Jenny is a female and NSSI is often a more acceptable behavior in females. Jenny's father is involved with her treatment, but he still does not believe she engages in NSSI or does not take it seriously as a concern in need of mental health treatment. He also has an authoritarian parenting style and restrains and punishes her for the behavior. This parenting style is predictive of ongoing NSSI. Additionally, it has been evidenced that having involvement from important figures in the family, such as a father, could help to prevent NSSI, treat, and maintain cessation of NSSI. Building a solid father/daughter relationship, in which her father is supportive and accepting of his daughter's need related to the self-injury, could assist her in her treatment. Jenny's father may also help her understand more about her cultural and ethnic identity so as she gets older, she will more holistically understand and appreciate her multiple heritages. A stronger parental relationship may support her in coping with future minority stress, which has the potential to exacerbate her NSSI behaviors.

Sam is a young, White male. His gender is the first, and one of the most prevalent, factors that appear to be influencing his self-injury. He injures in a way that is typical of males, which includes burning, wound picking, and punching. His forms of self-injury are consistent with what is seen in males and the gender role conflicts they may face. He also denies his self-injury, which again is common in males with GRC. If Sam is experiencing GRC, he could be even less likely to want to admit and seek help because NSSI is often viewed as a female issue. Instead of acknowledging his self-injury, Sam notes that it is just a way of "looking cool" to fit in with peers. Sam exhibits signs of depression, but it is difficult to determine if the depressive symptoms are a precursor of the NSSI or a consequence of the NSSI. Males often regulate emotions through the use of aggression, which contributes to externalizing disorders like depression. Additionally, the societal norms, stigma, and gender expectations that Sam faces in school could cause GRC, resulting in his negative emotional state and NSSI. Depression, anxiety, and isolation are highly inter-related with GRC. Sam has very little social support. Providing Sam more social support would have the potential to affect his restricted emotional expression and NSSI positively. His mother and the school need to get on board and find ways to increase Sam's support and help to reduce his isolation and bullying to mitigate his NSSI. Sam's mother wants to help, but she is not physically present enough in his life and does not know what parenting style would be best to help him.

Additionally, he has no clear male role model, which is a potential protective factor and could assist in modeling male behaviors that help combat stigma and GRC. Sam's teachers ignore the NSSI behaviors. In Sam's developmental stage, he needs to feel supported and form a positive self-concept. His teachers and mother are escalating the behavior by trying to ignore that it is happening, assuming that nothing is wrong if Sam is quiet and not aggressive. They are hindering his development of self by making him feel like he is less than and not worthy of attention. Sam is often the target of bullying and plays many violent video games. Violent experiences in males are known to lead to negative mood states, which is reflected in his interpersonal interactions and relationships with parents, teachers, and various others in a variety of environments. If his bullying is reduced in school and his teachers begin to notice him, he might be able to decrease his bursts of anger, ultimately reducing his time in detention and poor self-concept.

Lesbian, gay, bisexual, and transgender populations

There is some evidence that links acts of deliberate self-harm to marginalized sexual orientations and sexual minority stress with higher reporting among those who identify as lesbian, gay, bisexual, and transgender (LGBTQ+) (Almeida et al., 2009). Youth who identify as LGBTQ+, which is the non-dominant sexual group, are at an increased risk for NSSI as well as more frequent and severe NSSI behaviors, as compared to heterosexual youth, due to minority-related stressors (Fox et al., 2018). Similar to all youth, NSSI is linked to emotional distress, depression, anxiety, and low self-esteem, but sexual minority youth are especially vulnerable to NSSI and suicide, with rates as high as eight times more prevalent (Taliaferro & Muehlenkamp, 2017). Sexual minority stress includes discrimination, oppression, bullying, social isolation, microaggression, and prejudice, which all contribute to NSSI engagement, onset, and lifetime prevalence. Due to minority stress, sexual minority groups are also subject to higher levels of interpersonal and intrapersonal shame (DeCamp & Bakken, 2016). The shame is an indirect factor that could influence NSSI because sexual minorities may start to see themselves or their sexuality negatively. The bullying and discrimination may act as a direct factor, with NSSI used to cope with the emotional stress that the bullying and discrimination cause (Muehlenkamp et al., 2015). Those engaging in NSSI on the transmasculine spectrum (i.e., having a gender identity of a man, being male or a transgender man assigned female at birth, and/or identifying as genderqueer or non-binary) indicate that NSSI is affected by all of the following: gender nonconformity stress in childhood and adolescence, stigma related to minority status, identity development conflicts, and proximal minority stress from hiding their transmasculine status. NSSI is also affected by transgender identity development tasks, such as the exploration of new identity and the coming-out process (Jackman et al., 2018).

The case of Charlotte

In the case of Charlotte, she is a bisexual, non-binary female. As a non-binary (sometimes referred to as genderqueer) female, Charlotte recognizes she is a female but does not adhere strictly to the gender identity. She has androgynous or gender fluid qualities, both feminine and masculine. Additionally, she identifies her sexual orientation as bisexual, which means she is sexually attracted to both males and females. These two factors could cause Charlotte to experience GRC due to societal expectations regarding what is considered male or female. Identifying as non-binary often can confuse people, and it is still associated with mental disorders (which it is not), which promotes further stigma and ostracism for this population. This can cause stress and feelings of shame. She has already struggled in her cognitive development due to her sexual abuse, but further compounding this issue is her struggle with gender development and gender consistency. These internal struggles cause greater gender role conflicts and may likely affect her self-concept. Her sexual orientation is another source of minority stress. Being part of a non-dominant sexual group places her at increased risk for NSSI and more frequent and severe acts of NSSI. Sexual minority stress comes from many areas, such as stigma, discrimination, oppression, and prejudice. Charlotte's minority stress is dramatically increased due to the shame of non-disclosure to her parents. Telling her parents could reduce the impact of possible lifetime engagement in NSSI. Interpersonal and intrapersonal shame are much more prevalent for Charlotte because of her non-disclosure and having to hide her self-injury, sexual orientation, and gender orientation (DeCamp & Bakken, 2016). Facilitating connections with gender minority peers, seeking individual therapy, coming out to family, and creating a healthy self-concept and identity that is inclusive of gender and sexual orientation will assist in reducing NSSI behaviors for Charlotte.

Conclusion

There are many risk and related factors for NSSI onset and engagement. Cognitive developmental stages, along with gender, racial, and ethnic identity development, all have the potential to play an integral role in the lives of those engaging in NSSI. Given the context, each of these aspects can be a risk or protective factor for NSSI. Many differences exist between the ways males and females display and engage in NSSI behaviors. These differences stem from biological and socio-environmental contexts. They are critical to recognize when working with clients who self-injure because these factors can greatly affect assessment and treatment. Gender-related conflict must be addressed in order to help change the contexts for many male clients engaging in NSSI. Culture and diversity affect NSSI in a variety of ways. Feeling a sense of belonging within someone's racial and ethnic identity can affect their engagement in NSSI. More research needs to be conducted on culture, ethnicity, and race to fully understand how these concepts contribute to and influence NSSI onset and engagement.

TEXTBOX 6.1 REFLECTING ON YOUR OWN GENDER EXPECTATIONS

A clinician must be aware of how their own gender expectations play a role in the conceptualization and diagnosis of their client. Intersections of client gendered behavior and clinician gender expectations can affect clients, causing greater sources of stress. This is why it is critical to have a strong understanding of what gender roles and assumptions may consciously or unconsciously guide us. What gender role expectations do you have for males and females? How did your own upbringing affect your gender expectations? In what ways do you feel gender messages have guided you in choices in your own life (e.g., relationships, chores, careers, educational choices, etc.)? Are there things you consider for "boys" or "girls"?

REFERENCES

Almeida, J., Johnson, R.M., Corliss, H.L., Molnar, B.E., & Azrael, D. (2009). Emotional distress among LGBT youth: The influence of perceived discrimination based on sexual orientation. *Journal of Youth and Adolescence*, 38(7), 1001–1014. doi:10.1007/s10964-009-9397-9

Arnett, J.J. (2000). Emerging adulthood: A theory of development from the late teens through the twenties. *Am Psychol*, 55(5), 469–480.

Bandura, A. (1986). *Social Foundations of Thought and Action: A Social Cognitive Theory*. Englewood Cliffs, NJ: Prentice-Hall.

Barrocas, A.L., Hankin, B.L., Young, J.F., & Abela, J.R. (2012). Rates of nonsuicidal self-injury in youth: Age, sex, and behavioral methods in a community sample. *Pediatrics*, 130(1), 39–45. doi:10.1542/peds.2011-2094

Bem, S.L. (1983). Gender schema theory and its implications for child development: Raising gender-aschematic children in a gender-schematic society. *Signs*, 8, 598–616. doi:10.1086/493998

Blazina, C., Eddins, R., Burridge, A., & Settle, A.G. (2007). The relationship between masculinity ideology, loneliness, and separation-individuation difficulties. *The Journal of Men's Studies*, 15, 101–109. doi:10.3149/jms.1501.101

Breen, A.V., Lewis, S.P., & Sutherland, O. (2013). Brief report: Non-suicidal self-injury in the context of self and identity development. *Journal of Adult Development*, 20(1), 57–62. doi:10.1007/s10804-013-9156-8

Chesin, M.S., Moster, A.N., & Jeglic, E.L. (2013). Non-suicidal self-injury among ethnically and racially diverse emerging adults: Do factors unique to the minority experience matter? *Current Psychology*, 32(4), 318–328. doi:10.1007/s12144-013-9185-2

Claes, L., Luyckx, K., Baetens, I., Van de Ven, M., & Witteman, C. (2015). Bullying and victimization, depressive mood, and non-suicidal self-injury in adolescents: The moderating role of parental support. *Journal of Child and Family Studies*, 24(11), 3363–3371. doi:10.1007/s10826-015-0138-2

Claes, L., Luyckx, K., & Bijttebier, P. (2014). Non-suicidal self-injury in adolescents: Prevalence and associations with identity formation above and beyond depression. *Personality and Individual Differences*, 61, 101–104. doi:10.1016/j.paid.2013.12.019

Cohn, A.M., Jakupcak, M., Seibert, L.A., Hildebrandt, T.B., & Zeichner, A. (2010). The role of emotion dysregulation in the association between men's restrictive emotionality and use of physical aggression. *Psychology of Men & Masculinity*, 11, 53–64. doi:10.1037/a0018090

Colucci, E., Lester, D. (Eds.), Hjelmeland, H., & Park, B.C.B. (Collaborators). (2013). *Suicide and culture: Understanding the context*. Cambridge, MA: Hogrefe Publishing.

Crowell, S.E., Beauchaine, T.P., McCauley, E., Smith, C.J., Vasilev, C.A., & Stevens, A.L. (2008). Parent-child interactions, peripheral serotonin, and self-inflicted injury in adolescents. *Journal of Consulting and Clinical Psychology*, 76, 15–21. doi:10.1037/0022-006x.76.1.15

DeCamp, W., & Bakken, N.W. (2016). Self-injury, suicide ideation, and sexual orientation: Differences in causes and correlates among high school students. *Journal of Injury and Violence Research*, 8(1), 15. doi:10.5249/jivr.v8i1.545

Erikson, E. (1968). *Identity: Youth and crisis*. New York, NY: W.W. Norton & Company.

Erikson, E. (1993). *Childhood and society*. New York, NY: W.W. Norton & Company.

Fox, K.R., Hooley, J.M., Smith, D.M., Ribeiro, J.D., Huang, X., Nock, M.K., & Franklin, J.C. (2018). Self-injurious thoughts and behaviors may be more common and severe among people identifying as a sexual minority. *Behavior Therapy*, 49(5), 768–780. doi:10.1016/j.beth.2017.11.009

Gough, B., & Robertson, S. (2010). *Men, Masculinities and Health: Critical Perspectives*. New York, NY: Palgrave Macmillan. doi:10.1007/978-1-137-08076-9

Gratz, K.L. (2006). Risk factors for deliberate self-harm among female college students: The role and interaction of childhood maltreatment, emotional inexpressivity, and affect intensity/reactivity. *American Journal of Orthopsychiatry*, 76(2), 238–250. doi:10.1037/0002-9432.76.2.238

Gratz, K.L., Latzman, R.D., Young, J., Heiden, L.J., Damon, J., Hight, T., & Tull, M.T. (2012). Deliberate self-harm among underserved adolescents: The moderating roles of gender, race, and school-level and association with borderline personality features. *Personality Disorders: Theory, Research, and Treatment*, 3(1), 39. doi:10.1037/a0022107

Green, J.D., & Jakupcak, M. (2016). Masculinity and men's self-harm behaviors: Implications for non-suicidal self-injury disorder. *Psychology of Men & Masculinity*, 17(2), 147. doi:10.1037/a0039691

Hankin, B.L., Mermelstein, R., & Roesch, L. (2007). Sex differences in adolescent depression: Stress exposure and reactivity models. *Child Development*, 78(1), 279–295. doi:10.1111/j.1467-8624.2007.00997.x

Harter, S. (2012). *The construction of the self: Developmental and sociocultural foundations* (2nd ed.). New York, NY: Guilford Press.

International Society for the Study of Self-Injury (ISSSI). (2019). What is non-suicidal self injury? Retrieved January 3, 2019 from http://itriples.org

Jackman, K., Edgar, B., Ling, A., Honig, J., & Bockting, W. (2018). Experiences of transmasculine spectrum people who report nonsuicidal self-injury: A qualitative investigation. *Journal of Counseling Psychology*, 65(5), 586–597. doi:10.1037/cou0000304

Klonsky, E.D., & Muehlenkamp, J.J. (2007). Self-injury: A research review for the practitioner. *Journal of Clinical Psychology*, 63(11), 1045–1056. doi:10.1002/jclp.20412

Kohlberg, L. (1966). A cognitive-developmental analysis of children's sex-role concepts and attitudes. In E.E. Maccoby (Ed.), *The development of sex differences* (pp. 82–173). Stanford, CA: Stanford University Press. doi:10.1002/bs.3830130110

Kroger, J., & Marcia, J.E. (2011). The identity statuses: Origins, meanings, and interpretations. In: *Handbook of identity theory and research* (pp. 31–53). New York, NY: Springer. doi:10.1007/978-1-4419-7988-9_2

Kuentzel, J.G., Arble, E., Boutros, N., Chugani, D., & Barnett, D. (2012). Nonsuicidal self-injury in an ethnically diverse college sample. *American Journal of Orthopsychiatry*, 82(3), 291–297. doi:10.1111/j.1939-0025.2012.01167.x

Kwon, H., Yoon, K.L., Joormann, J., & Kwon, J.H. (2013). Cultural and gender differences in emotion regulation: Relation to depression. *Cognition & Emotion*, 27(5), 769–782. doi:10.1080/02699931.2013.792244

Landrine, H., Klonoff, E.A., Corral, I., Fernandez, S., & Roesch, S. (2006). Conceptualizing and measuring ethnic discrimination in health research. *Journal of Behavioral Medicine*, 29(1), 79. doi:10.1007/s10865-005-9029-0

Laye-Gindhu, A., & Schonert-Reichl, K.A. (2005). Nonsuicidal self-harm among community adolescents: Understanding the "whats" and "whys" of self-harm. *Journal of Youth and Adolescence*, 34(5), 447–457. doi:10.1007/s10964-005-7262-z

Messer, J.M., & Fremouw, W.J. (2008). A critical review of explanatory models for self-mutilating behaviors in adolescents. *Clinical Psychology Review*, 28, 162–178. doi:10.1016/j.cpr.2007.04.006

Meyer, I.H. (2003). Prejudice, social stress, and mental health in lesbian, gay, and bisexual populations: Conceptual issues and research evidence. *Psychological Bulletin*, 129, 674–697. doi:10.1037/0033-2909.129.5.674

Money, J., & Ehrhardt, A. (1972). *Man and woman, boy and girl*. Baltimore, MD: Johns Hopkins University Press.

Muehlenkamp, J.J., Hilt, L.M., Ehlinger, P.P., & McMillan, T. (2015). Nonsuicidal self-injury in sexual minority college students: A test of theoretical integration. *Child and Adolescent Psychiatry and Mental Health*, 9(1), 16. doi:10.1186/s13034-015-0050-

Nock, M.K. (2008). Actions speak louder than words: An elaborated theoretical model of the social functions of self-injury and other harmful behaviors. *Applied and Preventive Psychology*, 12(4), 159–168. doi:10.1016/j.appsy.2008.05.002

Nolen-Hoeksema, S. (2012). Emotion regulation and psychopathology: The role of gender. *Annual Review of Clinical Psychology*, 8, 161–187. doi:10.1146/annurev-clinpsy-032511-143109

O'Neil, J.M. (2008). Summarizing 25 years of research on men's gender role conflict using the gender role conflict scale: New research paradigms and clinical implications. *The Counseling Psychologist*, 36(3), 358–445. doi:10.1177/0011000008317057

Pederson, E.L., & Vogel, D.L. (2007). Male gender role conflict and willingness to seek counseling: Testing a mediation model on college-aged men. *Journal of Counseling Psychology*, 54(4), 373. doi:10.1037/0022-0167.54.4.373

Piaget, J. (1958). The growth of logical thinking from childhood to adolescence. AMC, 10, 12. doi:10.1037/10034-000

Plener, P.L., Libal, G., Keller, F., Fegert, J.M., & Muehlenkamp, J.J. (2009). An international comparison of adolescent non-suicidal self-injury (NSSI) and suicide attempts: Germany and the USA. *Psychological Medicine*, 39(9), 1549–1558. doi:10.1017/s0033291708005114

Schillinger, D.J., & Andover, M.S. (2016). Gender role conflict and non-suicidal self-injury. Paper presented at Conference: Convention for the Association for Behavioral and Cognitive Therapies. New York, NY. Retrieved from https://www.researchgate.net/publication/309566109_Gender_Role_Conflict_and_Non-Suicidal_Self-Injury/references

Taliaferro, L.A., & Muehlenkamp, J.J. (2017). Nonsuicidal self-injury and suicidality among sexual minority youth: Risk factors and protective connectedness factors. *Academic Pediatrics*, 17(7), 715–722. doi:10.1016/j.acap.2016.11.002

Tipper, J. (1997). *The Canadian Girl Child: Determinants of the Health and Well-Being of Girls and Young Women*. Ottawa, ON: Canadian Institute of Child Health.

Wang, S.J. (2010). *The survey and analysis on the factors associated with self-injurious behaviors among college students* (Unpublished master's dissertation). Taishan Medical School, Shandong, People's Republic of China. (In Chinese).

Welsh, L.A., Archambault, F., Janus, M.D., & Brown, S.W. (1995). *Running for their Lives: Physical and Sexual Abuse of Runaway Adolescents*. New York, NY: Garland.

Wester, K.L., & Trepal, H.C. (2015). Nonsuicidal self-injury: Exploring the connection among race, ethnic identity, and ethnic belonging. *Journal of College Student Development*, 56(2), 127–139. doi:10.1353/csd.2015.0013

Wester, S.R., Arndt, D., Sedivy, S.K., & Arndt, L. (2010). Male police officers and stigma associated with counseling: The role of anticipated risks, anticipated benefits and gender role conflict. *Psychology of Men & Masculinity*, 11(4), 286. doi:10.1037/a0019108

Whitlock, J., Eckenrode, J., & Silverman, D. (2006). Self-injurious behaviors in a college population. *Pediatrics*, 117, 1939–1948. doi:10.1542/peds.2005-2543

Whitlock, J., Muehlenkamp, J., Purington, A., Eckenrode, J., Barreira, P., Baral Abrams, G.,… & Knox, K. (2011). Nonsuicidal self-injury in a college population: General trends and sex differences. *Journal of American College Health*, 59(8), 691–698. doi: 10.1080/07448481.2010.529626

Yates, T.M., Carlson, E.A., & Egeland, B. (2008). A prospective study of child maltreatment and self-injurious behavior in a community sample. *Development and Psychopathology*, 20(2), 651–671. doi:10.1017/s0954579408000321

Yates, T.M., Tracy, A.J., & Luthar, S.S. (2008). Nonsuicidal self-injury among "privileged" youths: Longitudinal and cross-sectional approaches to developmental process. *Journal of Consulting and Clinical Psychology*, 76(1), 52. doi:10.1037/0022-006x.76.1.52

Part III

Ethics and treatment of non-suicidal self-injury

Chapters in Part II provide information concerning the various interpersonal contexts in which NSSI occurs as well as clinical perspectives related to the purpose of NSSI across the lifespan with regard to the intersecting issues pertinant to care. Issues related to culture, identity development, gender, and function of NSSI are included throughout these sections related to assessment, interpretation, and clinical determinations for treatment. Formal and informal assessment techniques are included as we discuss ways to adapt assessments per needs of the client. Case scenarios initially presented in Part I are introduced again throughout Part III in order to examine additional factors and information that would result from screening and assessment procedures specific to NSSI and other commonly co-occurring factors. Treatment approaches, context, setting, and ethical limitations will be addressed throughout Part III to fully conceptualize the complex nature of NSSI treatment.

7 Ethical considerations when working with NSSI

Kelly Emelianchik-Key and Mariah Dern

Two of the biggest challenges for clinicians working with clients who self-injure are always ethical and legal considerations. How do we ethically and legally keep our clients and students safe while also protecting their confidentiality? We already know that non-suicidal self-injury is different from suicidal ideation, but we also know that non-suicidal self-injury can evolve to include suicidal ideation. Confidentiality and informed consent needs to be addressed from a legal, ethical, and clinical practice standpoint, while also working in the best interest of the client. Maintaining this balance can be challenging for any clinician. Age of the client and setting make these conflicts even murkier and more complex. Confidentiality and the rights of minors who are self-injuring are very different when compared with that of an adult who self-injures. One of the first steps in any setting is to determine the amount of risk involved with regard to the severity of the self-directed violence. Confidentiality and safety need to be the primary concern, followed by the ethical implications and codes for various practitioners that differ by setting and profession. The decisions we make as professionals not only influence our clients, but they also have ethical and legal implications for other professionals working with them. The following chapter will explore how to keep those who self-injure safe, while adhering to pertinent ethical and legal standards, and creating a confidential environment for our clients.

School environment

The second leading cause of death in adolescents is suicide (World Health Organization, 2015), and self-injury is a risk factor for future suicidal ideation and completed suicide (Hawton & Harriss, 2007). As noted in Chapter 5, self-harm and suicide have several overlapping risk factors, which proposes that they occur along the same continuum (Kapur et al., 2013). Various settings are potential locations for prevention efforts, but schools have the potential to contribute the most widespread intervention opportunities due to their ability to provide resources for a diverse population of individuals at the time of typical behavioral onset of NSSI.

School concerns and considerations

The concept of social contagion and NSSI spreading through schools can often lead the administration to be hesitant about providing intervention and prevention programs for students. Schools also carry concerns related to disclosure and confidentiality, the risk of iatrogenic effects, duty of care, the safety of the student and others, and ethical and legal implications. School mental health professionals (SMHP) (e.g., school psychologists or counselors) are essential to the assessment of and intervention with youth who engage in NSSI, but teachers are critical for early identification, as students most often have trusting relationships with teachers and engage with them regularly. Recent research in the area has found that while universal training of all staff significantly improves knowledge and confidence regarding dealing with NSSI, it is not sufficient to improve the behavior and prevent suicide identification (Heath et al., 2011). All teachers should be trained on how to identify NSSI in students and the ways to address it promptly with confidentiality in mind to prevent some of the fears school administration sometimes has concerning NSSI prevention and intervention.

Additionally, all schools should adopt a school protocol for handling NSSI. Protocols allow for a shared language, a predictable set of standards, and a framework for operation. If you are a clinician, teacher, or administrator in a school environment and do not know of an NSSI or suicide protocol in your school, you may need to create one. Without a protocol, it can be easier to stretch the boundaries of right and wrong, which can end up putting students in harm's way or jeopardize any trust students have in their teachers or counselors. If there is no protocol in your school, talk to your crisis team (typically made up of trained professionals in the helping profession) to create a plan. If your school does not have a crisis team in place, your first step may be to talk to the administration about forming one. A protocol should include a description of roles for everyone in the school and a plan for everyone to consistently follow when a student is identified as actively or recently engaging in NSSI behaviors. The goal for this NSSI protocol is to provide predictability and consistency, while legally and ethically doing due diligence for students. Further information on how to create a school protocol is presented in Chapter 9.

After an incident of NSSI is reported in a school setting, a student is often referred to the first responder: the SMHP (i.e., school counselor, school psychologist, or school social worker). A recent study revealed that 92% of school counselors reported working with a student who had self-injured (Duggan et al., 2011). Unfortunately, school mental health professionals working with individuals who engage in NSSI also report low levels of NSSI knowledge and feel unprepared to effectively work with adolescents who self-injure (Duggan et al., 2011; Roberts-Dobie & Donatelle, 2007). Complex legal, ethical, and practice dilemmas for schools and SMHP add to this unpreparedness. A SMHP is faced with the dilemma of what to do with the student who has disclosed the self-injury. Practice-based challenges stem from how to work with the student who is self-injuring or whether the school counselor should work with the student engaging in self-injury or refer out to a community-based setting. But before getting to this, the SMHP must make difficult choices regarding ethical and legal implications.

Ethical and legal implications in schools

Legal and ethical ramifications of NSSI require the SMHP to deal with the legal concept of duty to warn and protect, which is the legal obligation that mental health professionals have to warn or protect people from known impending danger. For a list of duty-to-warn laws in the United States for mental health professionals, see the National Conference of State Legislature webpage (http://www.ncsl.org/research/health/mental-health-professionals-duty-to-warn.aspx). Here you can find out more information about the law in your state regarding the duty to warn. As mental health professionals, school counselors, psychologists, and social workers we have a duty or legal obligation that requires mandatory action or performance when there is the potential for client harm. For a SMHP, this duty involves protecting the child from danger and potential suicide risk (since we know that NSSI carries a strong risk for eventual suicidal ideation and attempts). This duty requires the SMHP to break a student's confidentiality *if* suicidal ideation is suspected. Confidentiality is the SMHP's promise or agreement to respect the student's privacy by not disclosing anything revealed during counseling, except under agreed-upon conditions. Those conditions should be discussed with the student before engaging with them, but if a crisis presents and the student is in immediate need of help, then it is the SMHP's responsibility to inform the student of the limits of confidentiality in developmentally appropriate language. SMHPs are obligated to take appropriate action if students engage in behavior that presents a clear and imminent danger to themselves and others.

Ethical codes for school mental health professionals

Both the American Counseling Association Code of Ethics (2014) and the American School Counselor Association (ASCA) Ethical Standards for School Counselors (2016) can influence the actions taken by school counselors, depending on their state certification or licensure standards and professional affiliation. School psychologists are bound by the National Association of School Psychologists (NASP) Principles for Professional Ethics (2010). School social workers are bound by the National Association of Social Workers (NASW) Code of Ethics (2017) and the School Social Work Association of America (SSWAA). Trust is a key component in all of the ethical codes and essential to confidentiality.

For counselors, trust between the counselor and client should only be broken with the permission of the client or in situations with legal or ethical justification (ACA, 2014). The ASCA Ethical Standards for School Counselors A.2. codes address confidentiality in school settings and require school counselors to have a principal obligation to the student while honoring the legal rights of parents and legal requirements to prevent foreseeable harm (A.2.e and A.2.F). School counselors have a duty to notify parents if the child is a danger to self or others and to minimize the threat. If notification is necessary, the student should be informed and involved in the process in some capacity (ASCA, 2016). School psychologists are held to a similar standard of confidentiality through Standard I.2.4, which notes information should not be shared without the child's parent's or guardian's consent, except when the child is in immediate danger. It also notes that student assent should be gained whenever feasible before breaking confidence to parents. School social workers' ethical codes (2015) guide them to appraise the responsibility to and welfare of the student. The responsibility includes confidentiality and should be contrasted with the responsibility to the family and the school, and the focus should always be on the best interest of the student and within the legal and ethical confines of the student's right to privacy.

As you can see within all of the various SMHP ethical codes, respect for confidentiality is essential when working with students engaging in NSSI, but it may warrant breaking confidentiality to ensure parents are aware of any ongoing and serious harm resulting from self-injury. SMHPs have a legal and ethical duty to be knowledgeable about NSSI, and they have an obligation to develop or provide responsive protocols to accurately assess risk and provide service and necessary referrals. SMHPs also must be the ones to determine if confidentiality needs to be broken, along with how and when to engage in telling parents and guardians. If there are no current protocols in place, then a SMHP should at least have a series of steps that they can work through toward developing a course of action that is ethical and within legal standards. These steps below are the most critical steps to ensure the student and school are all safe.

Ethical considerations in the absence of a school protocol

1. Identify: school staff and administration are trained yearly regarding what to look for when it comes to NSSI in their students. The first step to addressing NSSI within the school is to correctly identify students' self-injury, which can be difficult because most students hide evidence of their self-injury.
2. Respond: the SMHP can respond in a way that is empathetic, neutral, and compassionate. If the NSSI just took place, the student may need to be referred to a school nurse to evaluate the wounds to prevent the risk of infection.
3. Assess: the NSSI behaviors would need to be assessed for severity and the SMHP would need to determine if suicidal ideation is present. Assessment should include immediate danger to self, general severity, suicide risk, contagion risk, and prevalence in the school.
   a. *Low Risk:* the student has engaged in NSSI for a relatively short amount of time, inconsistently, and with little to no need for medical intervention. The student has positive coping mechanisms in his or her life and can easily substitute negative coping strategies with education and encouragement. The student trusts some individuals in their life and can go to them for support if they are hurting.

   b. *High Risk:* the student has consistently been engaging in NSSI for an extended period of time and needs medical attention to treat their wounds. The student struggles to identify positive coping mechanisms and is resistant to swapping out potentially unhealthy coping strategies for new, more helpful coping mechanisms. The student also either may not have a good support system or not trust their support system with their story.
4. Engage: if it is determined that the student is not suicidal, the SMHP can then determine how best to build a therapeutic relationship that includes engaging the student in discussion regarding external supports (e.g. telling a parent or caregiver about their NSSI). Defining when to notify parents/guardians of a child's NSSI is complex, and the SMHP should weigh the student's risk profile with relevant legal obligations.
   a. *Low Risk:* psychoeducation and regular meetings with the guidance counselor or support group may be encouraged, along with a conversation on the NSSI behaviors that includes the student's parents. If the student is of elementary age, the point person may need to notify parents without the consent of the student. This is not ideal, but the student's parents have a right to know and may be able to support treatment strategies at home, potentially improving effectiveness of school-based interventions.
   b. *High Risk:* the SMHP will work with the student on how to get parents involved immediately. Ideally, the student has some sort of control in this process and doesn't feel like decisions are being made for them, but with them. The point person will meet with the student and his or her parents to create a plan to get outside services such as psychological, psychiatric, or medical appointments scheduled as well as to encourage an atmosphere of support and trust between parents and student. It is possible that the student may need immediate intervention from specialists. The parents may have additional questions or needs that could be addressed with psychoeducation, support groups, one-on-one counseling, or encouragement from the SMHP. A follow-up should always be scheduled at the end of a meeting to assess progress. If the parent of the student does not follow through with getting their child the help they need, legal reporting may be necessary.
5. Educate: once the level of risk is determined within a student (which includes environmental factors such as age, state guidelines, etc.), the SMHP will make a plan with the student and provide education on NSSI. Additionally, students should be provided with materials that assist them in thinking about how to communicate their needs and feelings to others, including peers, in a way that promotes feels of safety and connectedness. Education is important, but may also cause the student to feel a sense of shame. Focus on the student's strengths and leveraging their strengths to influence their experiences with distress.

6. Refer: depending on specific state regulations, legal and ethical reporting will be done by the SMHP regarding the risk of the student. The student will be referred out for additional resources and a community-based therapist.

SMHPs should always be direct and make sure that they are asking questions in a compassionate and empathetic way. If the student does not want to open up, it is recommended to avoid pressuring the student, since NSSI already arouses feelings of shame and defensiveness, which could result in displays of anger or withdrawal. SMHPs should always work within their scope of practice, and if they are not comfortable working with the student regarding NSSI, then referrals need to be made immediately. SMHPs should act in legal accordance, but also in a responsible and ethical manner. In the event a student is at imminent risk for suicide, parents/guardians must be notified, and the student will require additional assessment and may need to be held in a hospital or psychiatric facility to assess the threat for the client's personal safety.

School counseling ethical decision-making model

Ethical decision-making models are a foundation of support and guidance to help clinicians make appropriate ethical and legal decisions in the best interest of clients. They often differ regarding the theoretical approach and framework for good practice (Cottone & Claus, 2000). Ethical decision-making models are widespread in the literature, but there is a clear guideline on ways to go about selecting one. ASCA (2016) published the Solutions to Ethical Problems in Schools (STEPS) as a model for school counselors in the Ethical Code for School Counselors. The model has nine steps, which are noted below. It provides a clearly defined approach for school counselors to make ethical decisions when faced with a dilemma. These dilemmas could include what decision to make with clients with regard to breaking confidentiality when they are low risk and self-injuring.

1. Define the problem emotionally and intellectually.
2. Apply the ASCA and ACA ethical codes and the law.
3. Consider the students' chronological and developmental levels.
4. Consider the setting, parental rights, and minors' rights.
5. Apply the moral principles.
6. Determine your potential courses of action and their consequences.
7. Evaluate the selected action.
8. Consult.
9. Implement the course of action.

The case of Sam: Ethical and legal considerations

You are the school counselor, and Sam has been referred to you because he had an anger outburst in class. You must assess Sam and find out what is going on. Your school has no protocol for self-injury, and no one has mentioned anything about Sam self-injuring. When you meet Sam and start talking with him, you immediately notice burn marks on his arms. You tell Sam about confidentiality and what his rights are as a student. It is clear that he is uncomfortable when you ask him questions, and at one point he picks at a scab. Sam acts aloof at first and doesn't seem to be attending well to your statements. As you gather more information from Sam, you start to suspect he may be self-injuring. You then say to Sam, "Wow—those burns look like they hurt, what happened?" He begins to open up, and he tells you how he did them himself. He stated that a friend thought they looked cool. You talk to him about how often he does it and ask whether he has ever needed treatment for his injuries. You assess Sam's risk, and you inquire about suicidal thoughts and behaviors. Sam denies suicidal thoughts, but does share that he is isolated and tells you about being bullied, but states, "no one cares, though." You ask Sam what he means, and he tells you how he has self-injured in school before, and he often gets bullied in detention, but no one does anything about it. You start to realize the NSSI is a problem for Sam and maybe even within the school since no one has ever reported any of this to you about Sam. This puts the school at great liability, and Sam has also been in danger struggling with NSSI for quite some time. His self-injury has progressed from headbanging and punching to cutting and burning. He also tells you that he has picked fights before on purpose, but once got hurt badly, and he has not done it since. You determine his risk is low. He states his mother knows about his self-injury, but not to the full extent. Sam needs some supports in place, and he reports how much of the time he is isolated because of his mother's work schedule. You consult with an ethical decision-making model to determine the next steps and to make sure you have thought of everything involved in the case. You also make sure to document everything along the way, and you follow the protocol below:

1. *Define the problem emotionally and intellectually*. Sam is struggling with being bullied at school and is very isolated. He is engaging in NSSI. He has trouble expressing himself in words, and when he gets anxious, he self-injures further. He seems very sad and distant as he talks with you, but eventually opens up as time goes on. He seems to enjoy engaging with you after a while and says you are helping him. His grades are slowly decreasing, but Sam seems very insightful once he starts to open up.
2. *Apply the ASCA ethical codes and the law*. According to ASCA ethical codes (section A.2), you have to inform Sam about confidentiality and what the limits to confidentiality are as a minor. Additionally, under ASCA code A.11, you must report any known instances of bullying to the administration in the school, as well as considering if Sam being left home alone so much could be considered neglect. Currently, there is not enough information to determine if it is neglect. Clearly his basic needs are being met, but there needs to be a discussion with Sam's mother about Sam requiring more support and engagement at home. According to sections A.6, A.7, and A.8, you have the responsibility to refer Sam out for additional

counseling services if you cannot meet his needs at school, but you also have the responsibility to get him involved with group work on campus that will help him with emotional regulation and to gain peer support. Specific NSSI groups are not recommended in schools, but there can be general groups that could promote Sam's socioemotional learning and coping skills. Under section B.1, you have a responsibility to decide if you want to report the NSSI to Sam's mother. Sam says his mother already knows. Possibly encouraging Sam to have a more detailed conversation with his mother about what is going on and the severity of the bullying and NSSI would be a good option. Per section B.2, you have a responsibility to the school. With this responsibility, you do not have to share with them everything going on with Sam, but you have a global responsibility to report that NSSI is happening within the school and to discuss adopting a protocol and having teachers trained on what to do if they notice a student injuring in school. You must advocate on behalf of the students to have the teachers trained properly on how to work with students engaging in NSSI. Legally, you are in a gray area of the law. There is no immediate risk to Sam to break his confidentiality, and it is up to you to determine how much to tell his mother.

3. *Consider the students' chronological and developmental levels.* Sam is in a developmental stage where social support is very important. Sam's developmental age is concrete, and he may believe you are breaking his trust if you tell his mother. There will need to be a clear conversation with Sam about what you think is required for him to succeed at school and at home. He should understand that you care and are there to help him, but you have a responsibility as a counselor to make sure that he is safe. Although he needs more support in all areas of his life, due to his developmental age, he may not fully understand what this looks like.
4. *Consider the setting, parental rights, and minors' rights.* It is not unusual for you to make a referral for one of your students to see a specialized mental health professional. Sam and his mother would benefit greatly from family counseling. You want to stress the importance of Sam getting additional counseling services outside of school and seeking family therapy. You let his mother know that there is only so much that can be accomplished at school, but you would like to connect with his therapist, so you can establish a plan of support for Sam at school that will help him reach his goals. You let his mother know what the limits of confidentiality are within the school setting and what her rights are as a parent, and you discuss Sam's rights as a student. Additionally, you communicate to Sam's mother that you are concerned with the amount of time that Sam spends alone. You make sure to document everything you discuss with her.
5. *Apply the moral principles.* Beneficence, nonmaleficence, and justice are the moral principles that need to be addressed. What is in Sam's best interest and what will need to be done in order to keep him safe? Moreover, what is fair for Sam in regard to his treatment at school by teachers and peers? It is not acceptable or just that Sam is injuring at school and getting bullied

and that these things are not being handled properly by teachers, staff, and administration.

6. *Determine your potential courses of action and their consequences.*
   a. You can choose not to tell Sam's mother about the extent of his NSSI and promote his autonomy and the decision he makes to keep this from his mother. You assessed for risk, and you determine risk is low. However, you know that Sam seems depressed and needs additional services. On top of this, he is often left home alone, which further puts Sam and you at risk if something were to happen. But you could assist on campus through groups and complete some sessions with Sam while monitoring his progress and doing an ongoing assessment to make sure things don't get worse.
   b. You could tell Sam's mother on your own and go against Sam's wishes. Due to the amount of time spent alone and his depression symptoms, you know that he needs more than what you could offer. You want to make sure his mother knows to further stress the importance of family counseling services. But with this option, you break Sam's trust, and he may not be willing to engage in counseling with you or another therapist due to this experience not turning out the way he wanted.
   c. You could talk to Sam and help him to understand why he needs to tell his mother about what is going on and ask him to take part in the conversation with you and his mother. You can leave it up to Sam to make the call of what he wants to share. You can let Sam know that this conversation will happen with or without his permission, but you would love for him to be involved and help make some of the decisions about what to say and how to work with his mother. Sam might still be upset, and rapport could still be broken, but it is a decision that he will have to make. You give him some autonomy over his own decisions.
7. *Evaluate the selected action.* You decide to tell Sam that you will be talking to his mother about the self-injury but would like very much for him to lead the conversation. It is important he have some autonomy, and with the lack of support in his life, you need to make sure that he gets additional support and services outside of school. Doing so sooner is better than waiting until later.
8. *Consult.* You talk with another school counselor about your decision and the option that you thought was best. You seek out supervision and support. Additionally, you consult with your school's legal department to make sure you are not overlooking anything regarding the law and your responsibility.
9. *Implement the course of action.* Sam wasn't happy initially with having to talk with his mother, but he did agree and led the conversation. You discussed it with him before you invited his mother into session and did some role-playing to help him. He appreciated that you practiced with him, and he was able to open up to his mother without getting angry at her.

Ethical tips for school counselors

The American School Counseling Association provides ethical tips for school counselors (https://www.schoolcounselor.org/school-counselors-members/legal-ethical/ethical-tips-for-school-counselors) to adhere to standards. Even though these tips are from a school perspective, many of them remain useful to all counselors working with children and youth, and we have adapted them to a broad base of settings.

1. Act in the best interest of the client.
2. Inform the client of limits to confidentiality as soon as possible, preferably before counseling begins.
3. Increase awareness of attitudes and beliefs. Our own values regarding NSSI, why children engage, and beliefs about suicide should not inform the process.
4. Understand diversity and cultural backgrounds, including your own diverse identity, and the ways it could affect treatment.
5. Function within your scope of practice and competence.
6. Fully explain what your role is, what you do, and your theoretical background.
7. Encourage family involvement with student permission.
8. Follow your job description and function, while maintaining your ethical codes. Be aware of where these two things could conflict.
9. Read the ethics and standards of your profession.
10. Consult with supervisors, colleagues, and other professionals when you need support to work in the best interest of the client.
11. Do not practice in isolation, and be part of professional organizations that will help guide practice.
12. Stay up to date with laws and court rulings, especially as they pertain to minors; additionally, anything that may be a state law vs. federal law.
13. Consult with a school district attorney when necessary in a school setting or with legal counsel when necessary for community-based settings.

Community-based settings and ethical concerns

Most mental health providers encounter self-injury. When working with youth in school settings, things like confidentiality and social contagion need to remain at the forefront to make ethical decisions. When working with minors in a community-based setting, the issues are similar to those found in school settings, which include privacy and confidentiality, the propriety of involving parents upon discovery of self-injury, risk assessment and management, and appropriate treatment. It is central to see youth as collaborators in the intervention process and to provide them with choices in regard to outcomes and next steps. Additionally, clinicians need to ensure respectful language and demeanor are being utilized to ensure effective practice (Walsh, 2012). Mental health providers in community-based settings that work with youth need to pay attention to similar issues as school providers but are not bound by ethics and laws that mandate school providers.

Confidentiality

The biggest challenge that differs when working with children rather than adults is determining whether to break confidentiality and if/when to notify parents or guardians of the behavior. According to the American Counseling Association ethical code B.5.b, counselors inform parents and legal guardians of their role as the counselor and the nature of the counseling relationship. A collaborative relationship should be set up with parents and guardians that is in the best interest of the child. Breaking confidentiality is not required unless the duty to protect exists, and parents need to know the information to protect the welfare of their child in accordance with the law. Very similar ethical codes surround disclosure of information regarding minors for psychologists and social workers. This leaves mental health professionals in a gray area when working with minors. The ultimate decision needs to lie in a counselor's ability to do what is in the best interest of the client. That being said, in addition to providing the appropriate risk assessments, if the risk is low, the context and environmental factors in the home need to be considered. If reporting to an unsupportive parent, who may be verbally and emotionally abusive with a strict and punitive parenting style, could make the situation worse for the child at home, then the risk of breaking confidentiality should not outweigh the benefits. There should always be a conversation with the minor client that includes them in each step of the process, no matter what decision you make. You want the client to have some control over the process and have their feelings recognized and validated as important.

Ethical considerations

Having a formal process or protocol in place to work with clients engaging in NSSI in the community and agency-based setting would be ideal, but often, this is not the norm. Here are some ethical considerations as you work with NSSI. Always assess for risk and function of NSSI. You want to make sure that your client is not high risk. As noted in this book, Joiner's interpersonal theory of suicide poses the argument that with the right conditions, continued engagement in NSSI will eventually lead to suicide attempts. NSSI can be viewed as a precursor for eventual suicidal ideation and attempts. Though related to suicide, most often NSSI is used as a coping mechanism to deal with strong and overwhelming emotions and may serve as an anti-suicidal function. As clinicians, our values and beliefs about self-injury and suicidal ideation need exploration. NSSI and SI often bring about strong reactions and can evoke feelings of self-doubt and confidence concerns in clinicians. Clients need to feel safe and supported by the therapeutic relationship. Confidentiality needs to be clearly addressed in the informed consent and be an ongoing process, especially since NSSI is interrelated with suicide. Clinicians need to be very clear about the duty to protect, and if clients present with self-injuries that are major health concerns that are left unattended to or develop suicidal risk, then these situations could lead to mandatory reporting based on the severity of these risk factors. Each conversation about confidentiality and duty to protect should be documented along the way. As noted above, if the client is a minor, there needs to be an open conversation about parental or guardian disclosure, but in a way that is empowering and that does not completely remove client control (if possible).

Assessment

A full assessment of self-injury should begin at intake or first disclosure of NSSI. Many formal assessments of NSSI could be used and have multiple functions (many are noted in Chapter 5). This, along with an informal assessment, will help build rapport with the client and assist you in gaining a full picture of the NSSI behaviors. Due to the interrelatedness of suicide and NSSI, there should also be a formal and informal risk assessment for suicide completed. Ongoing suicide risk assessments should be done as you work with the client to be sure that suicidal ideations or plans do not become present throughout the course of therapy. Each of the assessments that are done for NSSI and suicide risk should always be documented. In addition to assessing the self-injury and suicide risk present, clinicians should determine the client's readiness for change. This will help gauge the point that treatment should begin. Counselors should be knowledgeable about NSSI and practice under the competence of their profession. This includes seeking out supervision, conducting research, gaining consultative support from colleagues, and engaging in other methods that will improve clinical insight and skills. Documentation should be kept throughout the entire process, and each time that the clinician seeks consultation. If the counselor is not progressing in the work with the client and nothing has helped the therapeutic impasse, a counselor is responsible for having a dialogue with the client about potentially seeking out services from another provider that could help due to more experience or through specialized techniques. As an ethical clinician, it is imperative that you use theoretically based practices that have an evidence base, but also that you practice in a way that is culturally competent and considers all aspects of diversity inherent within clients.

Safety planning

Part of a clinician's ethical responsibility is to provide a safety plan for their clients. One component of the safety plan includes ongoing risk assessments to continually evaluate elevated risk and make sure the NSSI is not getting worse. Counselors must uphold their ethical principles. The ethical principle of nonmaleficence asserts that a clinician must do no harm to their client (American Counseling Association, 2014). In other words, how do clinicians invoke the least amount of harm possible to reach a beneficial outcome? In most cases, a beneficial outcome would be that the client would stop self-harming himself or herself, but in order to do so, the clinician does not want to create more chaos or possible trauma. It is possible, whether your client is a minor or not, that they may have a home life that is less than ideal. The clinician must do their due diligence in keeping their client safe but also must do it in a way that will not cause more harm to the client in the long run via condemnation or shame. It is important that through this process, and many others, the client not feel judged or shocked by how a clinician reacts; this reaction may leave the client feeling even worse than when they came into the office. The last thing the clinician wants to do is to accidentally damage the therapeutic relationship due to shock, anxiety, or discomfort with treating NSSI. Not every client who engages in NSSI should be hospitalized, so doing so in a rash matter with a low-risk client could be detrimental for his or her trust in process of therapy and could cause him or her to be wary of mental health systems going forward. It is the constant balance of weighing potential harm with potential benefits to ensure "no harm" to the client. It is a paradox that exists between promoting a client's autonomy and nonmaleficence.

Safety planning can also include an actual plan or map, so to speak, that is created collaboratively with clients. It notes the client's triggers, strengths, resources, supportive people in their lives, and coping skills, and it outlines a plan if the client becomes too overwhelmed with emotion and does not know what to do. These plans usually provide clients with resources as alternatives to injuring. Some clinicians use a "no self-injury contract," which requires clients to promise not to self-injure and we recommend against using these as they are potentially harmful and largely ineffective. Plans are usually signed by the clinician and client (and parent if it is a minor client). Plans that include replacement behaviors are also largely ineffective at reducing self-injury. There is no evidence that replacement behaviors work and can invoke feelings of failure or shame if alternatives are not used according to the plan, potentially causing a client to feel the need to keep secret their injurious behaviors (Hasking et al., 2015). It takes away their best strategy for regulating emotions, which is also sometimes an antisuicide measure. No-harm contracts are often drafted to reduce client NSSI behaviors and were once thought to minimize liability risk for professionals, which have not been supported by empirical evidence (Lewis, 2007; McMyler & Pryjmachuk, 2008; Walsh, 2012). Legally, some researchers and counselors believe that the use of no-harm or no-suicide contracts are actually forcing clients into a relationship that they are not ready for (i.e., giving up the self-injury), which can cause more harm than good. Furthermore, these contracts also put stronger legal liability on the onus of the clinician, who has signed a piece of paper indicating knowledge of the client's self-injuring or suicidal ideations, yet let the client leave without sending out for further assessment or hospitalization. Thus, the contract may put clinicians and clients at greater risk.

Legal implications

Duty-to-protect laws are pretty clear with suicidal clientele and less clear for a client engaging in NSSI behaviors. Many of you reading this chapter are mandatory reporters, where you may need to breach confidentiality if you become aware of abuse or neglect of any kind. There is a fine line between self-injury and self-abuse, but safety is the clinician's first priority. If the client is self-injuring but not suicidal, then confidentiality may not need to be breached. However, if the clinician has reason to think that even though the client may not be suicidal, they are capable of accidentally hurting themselves more than what they planned, then the clinician may need to breach confidentiality. In cases where the client is under the age of 18, parents should almost always be involved in the conversation; however, an ethical decision-making model should be followed in any case where a client is engaging in NSSI behaviors.

Ethical decision-making model

The American Counseling Association (ACA) has created a practitioner guide for ethical decision-making (Forester-Mill & Davis, 2016). Whether or not you are a counselor, this guide offers a useful process for making hard ethical and legal decisions, with clear steps that can be followed. This model is made up of seven steps to think about when working through an ethical dilemma. The steps are as follows:

1. *Identify the problem/issue.* In this first step to navigating an ethical decision, your initial hurdle is to narrow down the facts from fiction. Spend some time writing down exactly what you know to be true and separate it from what *could* be true. You may want to think through whether your hard decision is an ethical, legal, professional, clinical, or professional problem. Specificity in this step will help you better determine what to do in your next steps.
2. *Apply a code of ethics or laws to this case.* Now that you have determined the problem find your professional code of ethics, whether it be from the American Counseling Association, the American Psychological Association, the National Association of Social Work (2008), or the National Educator Association (NEA). You will want to look through your particular professional code to see if it directly addresses your issue. If your issue is not found in a standard code of ethics, then you should proceed with the rest of the ethical decision-making model to brainstorm for further solutions and to further implement a plan.
3. *Determine the nature of the dilemma.* In this step of the model, you will first want to consider the dilemma concerning the five ethical principles:

- *Autonomy*: addresses respect for freedom of choice, independence, and self-determination. The counselor should encourage clients to make their own decisions based upon their value system and not always depend on the counselor. Some may say that the goal of counseling is for clients not to need counseling anymore, which can happen with a healthy understanding of autonomy.
- *Justice*: addresses the principle of wanting to do what is right and fair, not necessarily treating all clients the same , but treating others in ways that they need to be successful. For example, this may mean seeking out specialized testing for a client to determine if they need additional services (they are not necessarily being treated the same as other clients, but rather with the necessary fairness they deserve).
- *Beneficence*: addresses the clinician's responsibility to do good for the clients. This may look like prevention or early intervention in some environments, or this may simply be a clinician who is proactive about client needs.
- *Nonmaleficence*: addresses the concept of not harming others. Harm can be intentional or unintentional; the idea is to reflect the practice of weighing potential harm against the potential benefits when making decisions for clients.
- *Fidelity*: addresses the client's need to trust a clinician for a therapeutic relationship to be beneficial. Trust can be built when a clinician keeps promises, honors commitments, and is consistent.

When referencing these principles, some may pertain to your ethical dilemma more than the others. In theory, all should be held with equal weight when determining a course of action. Your professional judgment should be taken into account when considering the ethical principles. Similarly, you will want to look at the current research and literature, as you are most likely not the first person to ask a particular question or to be in a certain predicament. Please do not try to reinvent the wheel if someone has already addressed this issue within a study or has the time, resources, effort, and experience to speak on the topic. It is time to consult your colleagues, other counselors, your supervisors, or other professional associations and organizations. The consultation you have with your colleagues will often illuminate, simplify, or clarify an issue that you are having with this ethical dilemma. As with other issues, having an outside voice to process with can be invaluable.

4. *Generate potential courses of action*. Now that you have determined the problem, gathered all the info you can find about the topic, reviewed what others have done in the past, and processed with your colleagues, it is time to brainstorm all possible outcomes. In this step, you will want to write down every decision you could make regarding this ethical dilemma and carry it through to the very end (making a visual decision tree may be helpful for some). Be sure to include the decisions that you are pretty sure will not work or that you will not choose. The idea is not to edit your thoughts, but just to brainstorm what *could* be.

5. *Consider the consequences and choose a course of action.* You can first look through all of the potential courses of action in the previous step and eliminate the ones that clearly do not seem to have desirable results or cause even more problems. Then, consider the rest by evaluating each option for all of the parties involved, including you as the clinician. In this step, you can determine if you even need to combine a couple of courses of action to create a desirable outcome. Which course of action seems to address the priorities in this ethical dilemma?
6. *Evaluate the selected course of action.* This step is here for you to consider if the course of action that you have chosen presents any new ethical dilemmas; it may be the best choice for this case, but does it open up another ethical can of worms? The ACA suggests that you ask yourself three questions in this step:
   - Assess your sense of fairness and justice in this situation. Would you treat others the same in this situation?
   - Ask yourself: if this situation got into the hands of the public, would you want your behavior to be reported in the press? Would you be okay with others finding out how you handled the situation?
   - Could you recommend this course of action to someone else in a similar situation)?

   If you can honestly answer each of the above questions with a "yes" and you feel this course of action is appropriate, it is time for the last step. If you cannot honestly answer every question with a "yes," you will want to start over in this process. You may not have brainstormed extensively enough, or perhaps you picked the wrong course of action and need to seek more counsel.
7. *Implement the course of action.* In the last step of this model, it is time to pursue what you have decided is the most ethical route for your dilemma. Be sure to take notes and document your process of how you got to this decision and what happened as a result of making this decision. The truth is that we do not always get it right. Humans are complicated, and as much as we would like to have all the information to make an informed decision, it's impossible sometimes. With detailed and accurate documentation of your ethical decision-making model, you will be able to defend your decision even if it does not go as planned. Success in some professions can look like making the right decision every time. Success in the helping field often looks like making the best decision you can with the limited information you have.

The case of Dean

You are a clinical mental health counselor in a small private practice. In your first session with Dean, you reviewed the meaning of informed consent and discussed the responsibility you have with the duty to warn and duty to protect. You also emphasized your responsibility to ensure his safety as a mandated reporter. In these first two sessions, you attempt to address the grief that Dean is feeling due to the loss of his partner. Dean avoids the conversation every time you circle back to grief. Dean would rather talk about sports or the weather. You have seen Dean four times before he tells you that his NSSI behaviors have increased along with his depressive symptoms. Dean jokingly states: "Dying might be more enjoyable than dealing with Parkinson's disease progression." You immediately address this with Dean and conduct a brief risk assessment with him for suicide, but he denies being suicidal. You also do a risk assessment of the NSSI behaviors and determine that his risk is moderate, given the circumstances surrounding him over the past year. You are not sure what the best course of action would be given that he denies suicidality, but his NSSI is lifelong, and his risk factors for suicide are moderate to high.

1. *Identify the problem/issue.* Dean clearly has suicidal ideation, but he is brushing it off. He has high-risk factors for suicide and is actively engaging in NSSI under the guise of trying to gain control over his spasms. You must determine if breaking confidentiality is necessary to keep Dean safe.
2. *Apply a code of ethics or laws to this case.* You refer to Section B.2.b. of the ACA ethical codes and re-read your responsibility to clients who have terminal illnesses. You note that counselors can choose what to do regarding breaking confidentiality when clients may consider hastening their own deaths in light of a terminal illness. You also check your state law and find that the law leaves it to the discretion of the therapist. Additionally, you read through the rest of section B regarding confidentiality limits, and you note that you must inform clients of their rights about confidentiality and its limits. You have done this already in your sessions with Dean.
3. *Determine the nature and dimensions of the dilemma.* You are unsure of what to do with Dean. You are responsible for keeping him safe, but he does not admit to active suicidal ideation, though he did joke about it. Additionally, he presents with many risk factors for suicide, such as depression, NSSI, the recent loss of a loved one, isolation, loss of faith, decline in health, refusal to adhere to treatment, incurable illness, hopelessness, and feeling like he is a burden. He admits to actively engaging in NSSI. You are torn between the idea that you must breach confidentiality due to your client's actions and possible suicidal thoughts. His Parkinson's disease also adds another layer to this complicated issue. It is an incurable disease that causes great discomfort and pain for some. The extent of his symptoms related to the Parkinson's is not yet fully understood. You respect your client's autonomy and his rights to make decisions concerning his health and illness. He needs to feel like he is in control, but you need to keep him safe. As a counselor, you have a responsibility for providing beneficence. You do not think his disease has progressed to a point where hastening his death is a viable option for him, although you know that this is not your decision to make. This is based on your own value system and what you know about ethics and the law.
4. *Generate potential courses of action.* (A) You could tell the client that you will be referring him for hospitalization to keep him safe. (B) You could continue

to work with the client knowing that he may have the right to end his life due to his medical state at some point and be okay with whatever decision he makes. You can let him know that you will not try to talk him out of whatever he decides. (C) You could refer your client to someone else because you do not feel comfortable with the level of intensity and a gray area this client has in his case. (D) You could explain your fears and concerns with the client and explain that you would like to do ongoing in-depth suicide assessment as well as an assessment of his NSSI behaviors. You can note that you have concerns for his safety and respect, while you validate his right to make his own health decisions. Additionally, you can ask him if he'd be willing to allow confidentiality to be broken by bringing in a friend he trusts to share his thoughts on NSSI and disease struggles. You can let the client know that this would be the best course of action to keep him safe, and if he does not agree, you will have to break confidentiality and get a further evaluation to assure his safety before continuing your work together.

5. *Consider the potential consequences of all options and determine a course of action.* (A) Breaking confidentiality and referring the client for hospitalization could completely break rapport with the client. He may never trust you or another therapist again. You can add to his situation and make things worse for him. (B) Engaging in a discussion about his end-of-life decisions seems too premature. You could scare the client away or upset him since he never said he was thinking about suicide or admitted to active suicidal ideation. (C) The client is coming back each week, so you are building some rapport with him. He is gaining something from coming to therapy. Referring him out because you are not comfortable with the gray area in therapy seems premature and that it would break the client's trust in you. You can seek out consultation and support as you continue to work with the client. (D) You could upset the client and risk rupturing the relationship with the client with this option, but if explained in a supportive fashion, the client may feel empowered that you gave him a choice. Additionally, he will be able to make his own decision of whom he wants to involve in treatment and how much he wants to share.
6. *Evaluate the selected course of action.* You want to double-check with your supervisor, so you consult and address these questions together:
   - *Assess your sense of fairness and justice in this situation. Would you treat others the same in this situation?* You and your supervisor believe that (D) is the best option and would give the client the most autonomy in his care. You also agree that being open with him and expressing your concern is the fair thing to do.
   - *Ask yourself: if this situation got into the hands of the public, would you want your behavior to be reported in the press?* You are confident that choice (D) is the best one and that if you document everything that you have discussed, this would be in the best interest of the client and has the least amount of negative consequences. Additionally, if the client says no to this option, you tried and can document that this was

the choice your client made, which led you to break confidentiality without consent.

- *Could you recommend this course of action to someone else in a similar situation?* Yes. This option seems the best fit for the situation. Regardless, heavy documentation and keeping the client safe are the top priorities.

7. *Implement the course of action.* You discuss your concerns with the client and explain the choice that you believe you need to make. You let him know that ultimately his safety is the most important factor, and if he is not willing to follow your protocol, then you will be forced to break confidentiality and have him referred to a hospital for a full evaluation to keep him safe. The client was relieved that you brought this up to him. He still does not admit to being actively suicidal, but he does need help. He agrees to allow his friend to come into a session, and he opens up about his struggles. His friend is upset that he did not tell him sooner, and they make plans to check in with each other every other day. Additionally, Dean realizes how much he has missed his church friends and faith, and he agrees to go back to church with his peer this week. You will follow up with Dean each week and do screenings every time you meet as a safety precaution.

Conclusion

In this chapter, we have reviewed the possible ethical and legal standards that many mental health professionals face with NSSI clients, offered suggestions for when protocols may not be in place, described an ethical decision-making model, and further applied that model to two case studies. There are very few dichotomous instances in the mental health field where a simple "yes" or "no" is always warranted. NSSI is an issue that demands we lean into the gray areas; as there will be demographic or cultural nuances to every case that can change the outcome of a situation. It is important to remember that throughout the process of considering ethical and legal matters, you should confer with other professionals and continuously document your decisions.

REFERENCES

American Counseling Association. (2014). *Code of Ethics*. Alexandria, VA: Author.

American School Counselor Association. (2016). ASCA *Ethical Standards*. Alexandria, VA: Author.

Cottone, R.R., & Claus, R.E. (2000). Ethical decision-making models: A review of the literature. *Journal of Counseling & Development*, 78(3), 275–283. doi:10.1002/j.1556-6676.2000.tb01908.x

Duggan, J.M., Heath, N.L., Toste, J.R., & Ross, S. (2011). School counsellors' understanding of non-suicidal self-injury: Experiences and international variability. *Canadian Journal of Counselling and Psychotherapy*, 45, 327–348.

Forester-Miller, H., & Davis, T.E. (2016). Practitioner's guide to ethical decision making (Rev. ed.). Retrieved from http://www.counseling.org/docs/default-source/ethics/practioner's-guide-toethical-decision-making.pdf

Hasking, P., Rees, C., Martin, G., & Quigley, J. (2015). What happens when you tell someone you self-injure? The effects of disclosing NSSI to adults and peers. *BMC Public Health*, 15. doi:10.1186/s12889-015-2383-0
Hawton, K., & Harriss, L. (2007). Deliberate self-harm in young people: Characteristics and subsequent mortality in a 20-year cohort of patients presenting to hospital. *The Journal of Clinical Psychiatry*, 68, 1574–1583. doi:10.4088/jcp.v68n1017
Heath, N.L., Toste, J.R., Sornberger, M.J., & Wagner, C. (2011). Teachers' perceptions of non-suicidal self-injury in the schools. *School Mental Health*, 3(1), 35–43. doi:10.1007/s12310-010-9043-4
Kapur, N., Cooper, J., O'Connor, R.C., & Hawton, K. (2013). Non-suicidal self-injury v. attempted suicide: New diagnosis or false dichotomy? *The British Journal of Psychiatry*, 202(5), 326–328. doi:10.1192/bjp.bp.112.116111
Lewis, L.M. (2007). No-harm contracts: A review of what we know. *Suicide and Life-Threatening Behavior*, 37, 50–57. doi:10.1521/suli.2007.37.1.50
McMyler, C., & Pryjmachuk, S. (2008). Do "no-suicide" contracts work? *Journal of Psychiatric and Mental Health Nursing*, 15, 512–522. doi:10.1111/j.1365-2850.2008.01286.x
National Association of School Psychologists. (2010). *Principles for Professional Ethics*. Bethesda, MD: NASP.
National Association of Social Workers. (2008). *NASW Code of Ethics Guide to the Everyday Professional Conduct of Social Workers*. Washington, DC: Author.
Roberts-Dobie, S., & Donatelle, R.J. (2007). School counselors and student self-injury. *Journal of School Health*, 77(5), 257–264. doi:10.1111/j.1746-1561.2007.00201.x
Walsh, B.W. (2012). *Treating Self-Injury: A Practical Guide*. New York, NY: Guilford Press.
World Health Organization. (2015). Preventing suicide: A global imperative. Retrieved from https://apps.who.int/iris/bitstream/handle/10665/131056/9789241564779_eng.pdf;jsessionid=33E7E07B817BA168ECEB022431DEEF77?sequence=1

8 Non-suicidal self-injury and suicide

Amanda La Guardia

The Centers for Disease Control defines self-directed violence as anything a person does intentionally that causes injury to self, including death (2018), and typically includes suicide, suicide attempts, and para-suicidal behavior. Non-suicidal self-injury is an act done without the intent to die but involves the intentional destruction of body tissue through cutting, scratching, burning, hitting, or other methods as a way of coping with psychological distress, in a way not culturally sanctioned (Whitlock, 2010). The DSM 5 offers a clear differentiation between NSSI and suicide attempts in order to identify associated diagnostic symptomology and severity of behaviors in a seeming attempt to address the lack of a clear conceptual understanding of self-injury among clinicians, which can result in imprecise behavioral estimates need for appropriate treatment of NSSI. Clinicians and researchers who believe self-injury is a para-suicidal or suicidal behavior can misreport NSSI as a suicide attempt (Trepal & Wester, 2007). There continues to be a lack of consensus regarding understanding of behavioral functions and traits associated with NSSI, which contributes to the ongoing misinterpretation of suicidal intent in relation to NSSI (Cwik & Teismann, 2017, McAllister, 2003). As suicide is one of the leading causes of death worldwide, affecting both young people, adults, and older adults, per capita rates increasing with age, it is understandable that mental and behavioral health practitioners may have heightened concern when any behavior is associated with or similar to suicidal behaviors.

What does the research say?

Longitudinal data indicate NSSI may predict suicidal behavior (attempts) and may be a better predictor of future suicide attempts when compared with all other associated risk factors (e.g., depression, psychosocial functioning, and prior attempts) (Whitlock, et al., 2013; Wilkinson et al., 2011). The interpersonal-psychological theory of suicide (IPTS) purports the idea that suicidal intent results from two interpersonal states that relate to a desire to end one's own life, but the desire itself is not enough for suicide (Joiner, 2005). An individual's capacity for suicide likely stems from repeated experiences with conditioned and painful events (e.g., self-injurious behavior) (Van Orden et al., 2008); thus, anyone is susceptible to circumstances that could lead to suicidal thoughts and behaviors due to the highly contextualized factors involved.

Suicide rates are highest among middle-aged white men, and despite suicide dropping off as a leading cause of death, it continues to be a significant health risk for adults. "In 2015, the highest suicide rate (19.6) was among adults between 45 and 64 years of age. The second highest rate (19.4) occurred in those 85 years or older" (AFSP, 2017, para. 2). Knowing population-specific concerns may help attend to stated self-deprecating thoughts and observed behaviors that are self destructive; however, knowledge of environmental and contextual factors that create barriers to perceived life satisfaction and happiness may assist clinicians in making difficult decisions regarding client care (Koivumaa-Honkanen, et al., 2001). Franklin et al. (2017) recently completed a meta-analysis of risk factor data across 50 years of research on suicidal thoughts and behaviors. His analysis of 365 published studies revealed that simple attention to risk factors, combined or otherwise, typically failed to predict individuals with suicidal thoughts and behaviors beyond chance in both general population and clinical samples. Specific to individuals engaging in self-injury, the meta-analysis failed to predict differences in suicidal ideation, suicide attempts, and suicide deaths when comparing groups engaging in NSSI who indicated prior ideation, attempts, or only self-injurious behaviors. While prior non-suicidal self-injury was found to be the strongest predictor of eventual suicide attempts across samples, it was not significantly different from other categories evaluated (e.g., prior suicide attempts), while prior psychiatric treatment history (specifically hospitalization) predicted death by suicide more than other risk groups. Franklin et al. (2017) hoped to highlight the need for more research regarding suicide and changes in the methodological and analytic approaches used to evaluate data, so clinically useful findings could emerge. An increase in studies on children and adolescents is also needed. Thus, the recommendation of these researchers was to continue to rely on current methods for risk assessment and clinical treatment decisions while researchers develop studies capable of analyzing suicidal thoughts and behaviors in a more nuanced, complex way to elucidate patterns or sequenced combinations of factors (algorithms) rather than isolated risk and protective factors.

Franklin (2018) discussed in a presentation at the American Association for Suicidology (AAS) conference a way of thinking about suicide that would align with patterned assessment or use of algorithms to assess factors contributing to suicidal thoughts and behaviors (STB) that may be more useful in understanding suicide. This complex way of analyzing suicidality may be more appropriate given the causes of suicide are often difficult to discern (not determinant across individuals or groups) and need to be considered within the context of broader psychological theory (within the context of the individual). Franklin postulates that suicide may follow with scientific theories of indeterminacy, which is an idea philosophically related to deconstructionism (i.e., an idea or construct, such as suicide, cannot be understood divorced from context). This means that the clinician, a peer, or family member would likely be the best person to determine if someone is likely to attempt suicide if these individuals understood the context of the person at risk (i.e., their needs, beliefs, and barriers) and were willing to consider suicide as a possible outcome related to that context. Following Franklin's logic, anyone could engage in suicidal behavior given certain, individually specific, circumstances. He encouraged clinicians to think about what would have to happen in their own lives that might lead them to think about suicide as an option and then reflect on the conditions that would need to exist for an attempt to occur. Then, given that self-reflective exercise, clinicians should think about what they would like to learn about their clients that might help them to understand better clients' unique context of risk.

The case of Dean

We could practice applying the ideas of indeterminacy presented by Franklin to the case of Dean; as a clinician, what other information might we need to know to further our understanding of Dean's risk for suicide? NSSI in itself is a risk factor for suicide, in addition to prolonged engagement with NSSI as a coping mechanism throughout the lifespan. Dean has experienced prolonged engagement with NSSI. Dean has also recently lost his partner, who was the only person he was able to confide in about his NSSI behaviors. Additionally, Dean is facing a debilitating and painful diagnosis of Parkinson's disease, which is currently incurable. Dean is consumed with fear of being unable to care for himself in the future as his illness progresses. For Dean, these factors may create the context needed to make it more likely for Dean to consider ending his life and making a suicide attempt. From what we do know about suicide and from suicide risk assessment scales (such as the SAD PERSON Scale), Dean would score high for suicide risk. As clinicians, we would want to use a formal scale to assess Dean's risk, but also engage Dean in dialogue that would help us to understand his distinctive framework for risk and access to means for suicide, as suggested by Franklin and others.

Ideation and attempt

Understanding the nuances associated with those who are considering suicide as an option and those ready to make an attempt can be clinically difficult. While the Interpersonal-Psychological Theory of Suicide helps us to understand aspects of this process (as they relate to belongingness, perceived burdensomeness, acquired capability, and ability to act), research regarding biopsychosocial factors can assist in conceptualizing what conditions (internal and external) might lead one to shift from thinking to action. May and Klonsky (2016) analyzed 27 research studies regarding this shift. Their analysis indicated that anxiety, post-traumatic stress, drug use problems, and sexual abuse history were elevated for those who attempted versus those who experience ideation, but not strongly so. May and Klonsky concluded that, while more research is needed to facilitate differentiation between these two groups, acquired capability for suicide may be a key factor that separates those who think about suicide from those who attempt or complete. Lack of fear or avoidance of pain can facilitate and support a resolution to attempt suicide, and this factor is evident in the literature on non-suicidal self-injury, indicating that NSSI may be a mechanism for acquired capability for suicide (Willoughby et al., 2015). Supporting this research is the 3-Step Theory (3ST) of suicide that provides an idea-to-action framework to assist clinicians in identifying how one would move from ideation to attempt. This model indicates a link between pain (typically psychological) and hopelessness that leads to action, potentially facilitated by lack of connectedness (indicating connectedness as a protective factor, potentially reducing or preventing ideation). The model and associated research also indicate that dispositional (i.e., pain sensitivity), acquired (i.e., habituation to pain), and practical (i.e., access to means) aspects of suicidal behavior seem to predict attempt history beyond current or past ideation (Klonsky & May, 2015). Thus, if one is experiencing pain and hopelessness, perceived pain is greater than their perceived connectedness, and this person is capable of attempting suicide, then he or she would be at the greatest risk for an attempt.

Further to the idea-to-action framework, O'Connor and Kirtley (2018) developed the Integrated Motivation-Volitional model of suicide, which serves to evaluate the process of the framework. They postulate that ultimately an attempt occurs when a person feels a sense of humiliation or defeat with no prospect for improvement or escape (feeling trapped), leading to suicidal distress. If this distressing process activates repeatedly, it is easier to access and thus suicidal distress becomes more salient, potentially leading to a negative cognitive bias, which may lead a person to see reasons for suicide more readily in daily life. However, to move from ideation to action, one would need to experience several elements, potentially including access to means, planning, exposure to suicide or suicidal behavior, impulsivity, endurance toward physical pain, fearlessness about death, visualizations of dying, and past suicidal behavior (e.g., self-injury or self-harm). For more information about the Integrated Motivation-Volitional model of suicide, visit: http://www.suicideresearch.info/the-imv.

The case of Dean

Returning to the case of Dean, if we consider IPTS, Dean may have an acquired capability for suicide and may perceive himself to be a burden to others. Acquired capability may be a determining factor for Dean as he considers attempting suicide (lack of fear). The further Dean's disease progresses, the more pain he experiences, and the more he continues to lose control, Dean may resort to self-injuring behavior, which further builds his capability for suicide. Dean is also concerned about the future if he is unable to take care of himself. This is a feeling of burdensomeness. The more Dean feels like a burden to those around him and loses control of his health, the greater the risk he poses for moving from suicidal ideation to attempt. Dean's protective factors have included his faith and church community, which once was a central part of his life. His connectedness to the church as a support system is something that a clinician would need to focus on as Dean may be interested in reconnecting with that part of his life, but may also perceive barriers to doing so that could be overcome through counseling. The church appears to be part of Dean's sense of belonging. In recently losing his partner, he may need to find a new place where he feels comfortable, like he belongs. According to IPTS, if Dean continues to avoid the church or continues to push away from communities or people he connects with, he may completely lose his sense of belonging, making his risk of suicide much greater. Using the IMV framework, Dean could make a suicide attempt if and when he feels a sense of shame, embarrassment, or defeat with no hope for improvement in regard to his health. For example, he may feel he has been gone from church too long to return, embarrassed regarding his absence and his emerging physical needs associated with his illness, or afraid of encountering memories of his partner for whom he is still grieving. This is why it will be critical for a practitioner to assess Dean continually for suicidal ideation and a plan as his disease progresses and distance from others persists. Additionally, the clinician will have to monitor Dean's Parkinson's symptoms closely, as his experience with them may present an important factor potentially leading Dean to consider shifting from ideation to a suicide attempt. If a clinician determines that a suicide attempt is imminent, the clinician will have to check their state laws and ethical models in order to determine the best course of action in their work with Dean since he will have engaged in end-of-life decision-making potentially due to his debilitating and incurable illness. Then it will be up to the clinician to follow their ethical codes and decision-making models to best support and protect Dean (which may include hospitalization). Issues of personal autonomy and progression of suffering make decision-making in this case complex, which only heightens the need for interprofessional collaboration with regard to Dean's overall healthcare and professional consultation when determining levels of care required for treatment.

Suicide assessment

Given the clear complexity of suicidal thought and action and the potential outcomes if a clinician were to miss signs of suicide, assessment can seem daunting. While multiple assessment methods exist for evaluating risk, the Collaborative Assessment and Management of Suicidality (CAMS) approach is a widely accepted and highly research method for evaluating risk and developing appropriate treatment options for suicide. Key aspects of this approach align quite clearly with counseling perspectives in that one is encouraged to approach the topic of suicide non-judgmentally and empathically to understand a client's struggle related to suicide from the client's perspective. While this approach may sound simple, it can sometimes be difficult for professionals to discuss suicide as an option and honor a client's reasoning concerning their decision to potentially end her or his own life. Several approaches to suicide intervention also include the stance that clinicians, or indeed anyone, should broach suicide from a perspective of understanding or wanting to know more about the story that has led someone to consider suicide (e.g., Applied Suicide Intervention Skills Training or ASIST, Zero Suicide, and Suicide to Hope). The CAMS is an evidence-based assessment and treatment process for suicide intervention that is designed to facilitate the improvement of suicidal symptomology in an outpatient setting via a brief intervention format in a way that honors and elicits the client's story. Specialized training in CAMS is required to implement the process appropriately with clients. However, the CAMS Suicide Status Form-4 (SSF-4) is readily available online and is used for initial session assessment and follow-up care. For more on CAMS, visit: https://cams-care.com/about-cams/.

Linked to any suicide intervention is the need for assessment of access to lethal means. This assessment is an essential step to any suicide risk determination. Counseling on Access to Lethal Means, or CALM, is an established and well-researched approach. In order to make treatment decisions, build effective safety plans, and determine the level of care needed for suicide prevention, knowledge and reduction of access to lethal means can be the difference between life and death. Reducing access to lethal means is an evidence-based approach to reducing deaths by suicide for those at risk of suicidal behavior. Reducing access to means is thus an important component of any safety plan you develop with a client and/or the client's family. Free CALM training is available online at https://training.sprc.org/enrol/index.php?id=20 through the Suicide Prevention Resource Center.

Multiple useful inventories exist that can supplement any assessment process with a potentially suicidal client. The following have demonstrated sound validity and reliability for clinical use:

- Reasons for Living Inventory (S/RFLI; Linehan et al., 1983; Garza & Cramer, 2011)
- Interpersonal Needs Questionnaire (INQ; Van Orden et al., 2008, 2012)
- Acquired Capability for Suicide Questionnaire (ACSS/ACSS-FAD; Ribeiro et al., 2013)
- Suicidal Behaviors Questionnaire-Revised (SBQ-R; Osman et al., 2001)
- Beck Scale for Suicidal Ideation (BSS; Beck & Steer, 1991)
- Columbia Suicide Severity Rating Scale (C-SSRS; Posner et al., 2011; see http://cssrs.columbia.edu/the-columbia-scale-c-ssrs/about-the-scale/)

It is important to make note of assessments used and the clinical decision-making process utilized regarding determinations for level of care as well as resultant actions taken with clients within formal clinical treatment documentation. This is so you can link any clinical decisions regarding the level of care and treatment to sound, evidence-based assessment procedures grounded in theories of suicide. When working with any high-risk client, appropriate documentation is critical for continuity of care and assists in guarding against malpractice.

Levels of care

A stepped care approach to suicide prevention is a model prevalent in a variety of intervention programs and techniques, including the CAMS (Jobes et al., 2018). Stepped care methods advocate for the use of the least restrictive method for suicide prevention concerning the treatment and care of suicidal individuals from a person-centered (or patient-centric), systems approach. These steps move from the least restrictive, most cost-efficient methods, which may include peer intervention (in school systems), self-help strategies, support groups, or engagement with paraprofessionals, through to the most restrictive, costly methods (hospitalization). The CAMS is useful at every stage involving professional intervention including those working at crisis care hotlines up through those working at in-patient facilities. As a person becomes less psychologically stable and it has been identified that lethal means are accessible and difficult to remove or restrict, a person's safety needs are more likely to be met through increased levels or more restrictive levels of care. Ultimately, care should be determined based on an individual's immediate intrapersonal needs, need for support, and for clinical treatment. For more about levels of care and the Zero Suicide initiative, visit: http://zerosuicide.sprc.org/toolkit/treat/providing-least-restrictive-care.

Interprofessional collaboration

The Suicide Prevention Resource Center (SPRC) advocates for collaboration between health and mental health professionals when working with suicidal individuals. For suicidal individuals to receive effective care and treatment, professionals must "Promote the integration of primary care and behavioral health care to increase access to behavioral health services in primary care settings," (SPRC, 2019, p. 2) as often primary care is engaged prior to or in lieu of mental health services. Ultimately, it is important for you to know your role concerning client care, your level of responsibility concerning care, and your contribution to collaborative treatment with other health and behavioral/mental health professionals. Interprofessional Education Collaborative (IPEC) developed a set of competencies to assist professionals in working together for client care. These competencies emphasize teamwork, communication, interprofessional values and ethics, and knowledge of roles and responsibilities (IPEC, 2016). In order to act competently, you will need to reflect on the limitations of your knowledge and skills with regard to suicide prevention, intervention, and postvention (intervention after a suicide) and how you can facilitate the involvement of collaborators to complement your strengths and address gaps in your knowledge or limits in your role/scope of practice. You are not alone in preventing suicide. You are part of a community of care that includes the client, their family and friends, colleagues, and other professionals.

NSSI links to suicide

Non-suicidal self-injury often continues to be a problem among those who used the behavior in adolescence and received inadequate or no treatment to address it. Several cases reviewed in this text include contextual factors that could increase the risk for suicide or lead a clinician to react to NSSI as an act with suicidal intent (i.e., para-suicide or suicide attempt). Behaviors increase the risk of suicide more than thoughts. If a counselor interprets NSSI as a preparatory behavior or if the NSSI occurs as a method for interrupting an attempt, clinical concern regarding eventual suicide may be warranted within the context of acquired capability and the motivational-volitional model. However, assessment of NSSI as a preparatory behavior or method of interruption can be difficult to discern, making treatment determinations potentially more difficult. To simplify treatment decisions, it is important to note that many of the same interventions shown to be effective in the prevention of suicide have also demonstrated effectiveness in the treatment of NSSI (e.g., Dialectical Behavioral Therapy). Thus, the utilization of an overlapping approach focused on the functions of self-injury could serve a dual purpose. Use of evidence-based approaches in the treatment of both NSSI and suicide may be especially useful for clients with a suicide attempt history engaging in frequent NSSI, using a number of methods, and reporting lessened pain experience; these factors are associated with increased risk for suicide (Ammerman et al., 2015) and the inability to regulate distress (Nock & Mendes, 2008). Ultimately, NSSI itself has been linked to significantly greater risk of suicide attempt (Ribeiro et al., 2016), but considered alone, NSSI does not serve to increase odds of an attempt significantly on a practical level. Intervention with individuals engaging in NSSI may prove to be a useful suicide prevention strategy and assist in the cessation of the behavior itself.

Some key differences observed between non-clinical adolescents engaging in NSSI and their non-NSSI peers include depressive symptoms, suicidal ideation, hopelessness, body dissatisfaction, disordered eating, lack of peer and parental support, and lower self-esteem (Brausch & Gutierrez, 2010). It is important to note that recent research has indicated when working with clients who engage in eating-disordered behavior, the presence of self-injury can differentiate those thinking about suicide from those who might attempt (Pérez et al., 2018). Those with eating-disordered behaviors are at heightened risk for NSSI (Dodd et al., 2018). When thinking about treatment considerations for those engaging in NSSI and eating disordered behavior, it may be helpful to review the "Case of Charlotte" in Chapter 2 of this book. NSSI commonly co-occurs with other issues, like eating-disordered (ED) behaviors. In the "Case of Jimmy" in Chapter 3, Jimmy struggles with alcohol and substance misuse. NSSI often co-occurs with substance abuse/misuse (SA). For those with eating-disordered behaviors or for those engaging in substance abuse and misuse along with NSSI, impulsivity and control are all key factors in need of attention during treatment. Thus, clinicians need to consider core concerns (such as impulsivity) related to as many intersecting behavioral issues as possible to target underlying functions or influences.

Negative affect or internalized negative self-perception and perceptions of others are essential components related to NSSI, suicide, and other self-harming behaviors, such as ED and SA. Interpersonal stressors like criticism and experiences of social rejection can increase the urge to self-injure for those already engaging in the behavior. Internalized negative affect may increase the risk of suicide for individuals using NSSI to cope (Victor et al., 2018). Thus, emotional regulation likely plays a key role in the treatment of NSSI and prevention of suicide for individuals actively engaging in NSSI behaviors (Brausch & Woods, 2018).

Issues pertaining to emotional dysregulation are prevalent throughout the lifespan and intersect greatly with observations of emotional regulation during childhood (family of origin) as observed and experienced through caregiver conflict resolution, child-parent interactions, and, later, peer relationships. Skill deficits regarding the ability to self-soothe and tolerate emotional distress can be a common issue, especially among children and adolescents. These skill deficits have been linked to a lack of theory of mind skills (the inability to accurately perceive and interpret the emotional state of others) in aggressive children (Stellwagen & Kerig, 2018) and could be linked to the perception of interpersonal stressors. Thus, the teaching of empathy or empathic reaction to the distress of others, particularly in childhood, may assist with the development of skills associated with healthy emotional regulation. Within the "Case of Rick," approaching him in a way that communicates and models empathy will be critical. He needs to understand his emotions and how to convey them to others appropriately. Rick lacks adult relationships that are consistent, nurturing, and supportive in healthy ways.

Safety planning

Safety or stabilization planning requires involvement, investment, and agreement from the client and those involved in keeping the client safe (when short-term monitoring is necessary). Many versions of safety plans are available from a variety of sources, and examples are available in this book (see Appendix 12B). When writing a safety plan, it is useful to include some things, whether a practitioner designs the plan to prevent suicide or non-suicidal self-injury. Listing strengths and assets, useful and effective coping strategies for distress, and people who might be useful to contact when the client is feeling isolated or having self-deprecating thoughts are helpful in both in-session treatment and practice of healthy ways of being outside of session. The CAMS stabilization plan also suggests discussing how to reduce access to lethal means, the inclusion of emergency contact numbers (including the national suicide hotline

1-800-273-TALK), and potential barriers and solutions to attending scheduled treatment appointments. In safety planning, some issues come up regarding the right to die and client autonomy, especially when working with individuals who are terminally ill or are at the end of life.

Richards (2017) presents the rationalizations and justifications of patients seeking assisted suicide and their beliefs as well as their decisions to die. Typically, lawful assisted suicide is completed with the help of a doctor in countries or states where this practice is legally supported. Overall, participants believed, based on evidence, that physician-assisted suicide would be painless and similar to a "natural death," and the idea of having shared responsibility with a professional made the decision easier to justify and accept, while some simply wanted the power of the physician to ensure their death would happen in the way they wanted. Richards concluded that a person's social conditions influence the way in which they experience their illness, potentially linked to concepts like belongingness and burdensomeness. Many clinicians and researchers call for more focus on palliative care rather than the development of the practice of assisted suicide. However, at this point, suicide prevention is most certainly a duty for any behavioral health or health care professional and is mandated by a number of laws in many countries, including the United States (see https://www.treatmentadvocacycenter.org/storage/documents/Standards_-_The_Text-_June_2011.pdf for more information on standards for treatment in the United States). Autonomy and the practitioner's role in ensuring safety are constant struggles for those of us working with clients considering suicide or engaging in self-injury. Awareness of policy standards in your place of work, ethical standards within your profession, and the regulatory mandates of your license to practice will help guide your decisions. Client autonomy can present many gray areas in which difficult decisions must be made. I hope that the information in this book can assist you in reflecting on your own role as a counselor or health practitioner as you make the hard decisions we are called to make as part of our work within our respective communities.

REFERENCES

AFSP. (2017). About suicide: Suicide statitistics. Retrieved from https://afsp.org/about-suicide/suicide-statistics/

Ammerman, B.A., Burke, T.A., Alloy, L.B., & McCloskey, M.S. (2015). Subjective pain during NSSI as an active agent in suicide risk. *Psychiatry Research*, 236, 80–85. doi:10.1016/j.psychres.2015.12.028

Beck, A.T., & Steer, R.A. (1991). BSI, Beck scale for suicide ideation: Manual. San Antonio, TX: Psychological Corp.

Brausch, A.M., & Gutierrez, P.M. (2010). Differences in non-suicidal self-injury and suicide attempts in adolescents. *Journal of Youth and Adolescence*, 39(3), 233–242. doi:10.1007/s10964-009-9482-0

Brausch, A.M., & Woods, S.E. (2018). Emotion regulation deficits and nonsuicidal self-injury prospectively predict suicide ideation in adolescents. *Suicide & Life-Threatening Behavior*, 49(3), 868–880. doi:10.1111/sltb.12478

Centers for Disease Control and Prevention. (June 22, 2018). *Self-directed violence and other forms of self-injury*. Retrieved from https://www.cdc.gov/ncbddd/disabilityandsafety/self-injury.html

Cwik, J.C., & Teismann, T. (2017). Misclassification of self-directed violence. *Clinical Psychology & Psychotherapy*, 24(3), 677–686. doi:10.1002/cpp.2036

Dodd, D.R., Smith, A.R., Forrest, L.N., Witte, T.K., Bodell, L., Bartlett, M., … Goodwin, N. (2018). Interoceptive deficits, nonsuicidal self-injury, and suicide attempts among women with eating disorders. *Suicide and Life-Threatening Behavior*, 48(4), 438–448. doi:10.1111/sltb.12383

Franklin, J.C. (April 20, 2018). *All Our Data Are Pointing toward a Radically Different Paradigm for Suicide Research*. Washington, DC: American Association for Suicidology.

Franklin, J.C., Ribeiro, J.D., Fox, K.R., Bentley, K.H., Kleiman, E.M., Huang, X., … Nock, M.K. (2017). Risk factors for suicidal thoughts and behaviors: A meta-analysis of 50 years of research. *Psychological Bulletin*, 143(2), 187–232. doi:10.1037/bul0000084

Garza, M.J., & Cramer, R.J. (2011). The Spanish Reasons for Living Inventory (SRFL-I): Factor structure and association with suicide risk among Spanish speaking Hispanics. *Archives of Suicide Research*, 15(4), 354–371. doi:10.1080/13811118.2011.615704

Interprofessional Education Collaborative. (2016). *Core Competencies for Interprofessional Collaborative Practice: 2016 Update*. Washington, DC: Interprofessional Education Collaborative.

Jobes, D.A., Gregorian, M.J., & Colborn, V.A. (2018). A stepped care approach to clinical suicide prevention. *Psychological services*, 15(3), 243. doi:10.1037/ser0000229

Joiner, T.E. (2005). *Why people die by suicide*. Cambridge, MA: Harvard University Press.

Klonsky, E.D., & May, A.M. (2015). The Three-Step Theory (3ST): A new theory of suicide rooted in the "Ideation-to-Action" framework. *International Journal of Cognitive Therapy*, 8(Special Issue), 114–129. doi:10.1521/ijct.2015.8.2.114 or see https://www2.psych.ubc.ca/~klonsky/publications/3ST.pdf

Linehan, M.M., Goodstein, J.L., Nielsen, S.L., & Chiles, J.A. (1983). Reasons for staying alive when you are thinking of killing yourself: The Reasons for Living Inventory. *Journal of Consulting and Clinical Psychology*, 51(2), 276–286. doi: 10.1037/0022-006X.51.2.276

May, A.M., & Klonsky, E.D. (2016). What distinguishes suicide attempters from suicide ideators? A meta-analysis of potential factors. *Clinical Psychology: Science and Practice*, 23(1), 5–20. doi:10.1111/cpsp.12136

McAllister, M. (2003). Multiple meaning of self harm: A critical review. *International Journal of Mental Health Nursing*, 12(3), 177–185. doi:10.1046/j.1440-0979

Nock, M.K., & Mendes, W.B. (2008). Physiological arousal, distress tolerance, and social problem-solving deficits among adolescent self-injurers. *Journal of Consulting and Clinical Psychology*, 76(1), 28–38. doi:10.1037/0022-006X.76.1.28

O'Connor, R.C., & Kirtley, O.J. (2018). The integrated motivational-volitional model of suicidal behaviour. *Philosophical Transactions of the Royal Society B*, 373. doi:10.1098/rstb.2017.0268

Osman, A., Bagge, C.L., Gutierrez, P.M., Konick, L.C., Kopper, B.A., & Barrios, F.X. (2001). The Suicidal Behaviors Questionnaire-Revised (SBQ-R): Validation with clinical and nonclinical samples. *Assessment*, 8(4), 443–454. doi:10.1177/107319110100800409

Pérez, S., Ros, M.C., Folgado, J.E.L., & Marco, J.H. (2018). Non-suicidal self-injury differentiates suicide ideators and attempters and predicts future suicide attempts in patients with eating disorders. *Suicide & Life-Threatening Behavior*, doi:10.1111/sltb.12521

Posner, K., Brown, G.K., Stanley, B., Brent, D.A., Yershova, K.V., Oquendo, M.A., … Mann, J.J. (2011). The Columbia-Suicide Severity Rating Scale: Initial validity and internal consistency findings from three multisite studies with adolescents and adults. *The American journal of psychiatry*, 168(12), 1266–1277. doi:10.1176/appi.ajp.2011.10111704
Ribeiro, J.D., Bodell, L.P., Hames, J.L., Hagan, C.R., & Joiner, T.E. (2013). An empirically based approach to the assessment and management of suicidal behavior. *Journal of Psychotherapy Integration*, 23(3), 207–221. doi:10.1037/a0031416
Ribeiro, J.D., Franklin, J.C., Fox, K.R., Bentley, K.H., Kleiman, E.M., … Nock, M.K. (2016). Self-injurious thoughts and behaviors as risk factors for future suicide ideation, attempts, and death: A meta-analysis of longitudinal studies. *Psychological Medicine*, 46(2), 225–236. doi:10.1017/S0033291715001804
Richards, N. (2017). Assisted suicide as a remedy for suffering? The end-of-life preferences of British "suicide tourists". *Medical Anthropology*, 36(4), 348. doi:10.1080/01459740.2016.1255610
Stellwagen, K.K., & Kerig, P.K. (2018). Theory of mind deficits and reactive aggression in child psychiatric inpatients: Indirect effects through emotion dysregulation. *Journal of Child and Family Studies*, 27(10), 3385–3394. doi:10.1007/s10826-018-1161-x
SPRC. (2019). Suicide Prevention Resource Center: Effective care and treatment. Retrieved from https://www.sprc.org/comprehensive-approach/effective-care
Trepal, H.C., & Wester, K.L. (2007). Self-injurious behaviors, diagnoses, and treatment methods: What mental health professionals are reporting. *Journal of Mental Health Counseling*, 29(4), 363–375.
Van Orden, K.A., Witte, T.K., Gordon, K.H., Bender, T.W., & Joiner, T.E. (2008). Suicidal desire and the capability for suicide: Tests of the interpersonal-psychological theory of suicidal behavior among adults. *Journal of Consulting and Clinical Psychology*, 76, 72–83.
Van Orden, K.A., Cukrowicz, K.C., Witte, T.K., & Joiner, T.E. (2012). Thwarted belongingness and perceived burdensomeness: Construct validity and psychometric properties of the Interpersonal Needs Questionnaire. *Psychological Assessment*, 24(1), 197–215. doi:10.1037/a0025358
Victor, S.E., Scott, L.N., Stepp, S.D., & Goldstein, T.R. (2018). I want you to want me: Interpersonal stress and affective experiences as within-person predictors of nonsuicidal self-injury and suicide urges in daily life. *Suicide & Life-Threatening Behavior*, doi:10.1111/sltb.12513
Whitlock, J. (2010). What is self-injury? [Fact sheet] Cornell Research Program on Self-Injurious Behavior in Adolescents and Young Adults. Retrieved from http://www.selfinjury.bctr.cornell.edu/factsheet_aboutsi.asp
Whitlock, J., Meuhlenkamp, J., Eckenrode, J., Purington, A., Baral Abrams, G., Barreira, P., & Kress, V. (2013). Nonsuicidal self-injury as a gateway to suicide. *Journal of Adolescent Health*, 52(4), 486–492. doi:10.1016/j.jadohealth.2012.09.010
Wilkinson, P., Kelvin, R., Roberts, C., Dubicka, B., & Goodyer, I. (2011). Clinical and psychosocial predictors of suicide attempts and nonsuicidal self-injury in the Adolescent Depression Antidepressants and Psychotherapy Trial (ADAPT). *American Journal of Psychiatry*, 168(5), 495–501. doi:10.1176/appi.ajp.2010.10050718
Willoughby, T., Heffer, T., & Hamza, C.A. (2015). The link between nonsuicidal self-injury and acquired capability for suicide: A longitudinal study. *Journal of Abnormal Psychology*, 124(4), 1110–1115. doi:10.1037/abn0000104

9 Prevention and treatment strategies in educational settings

Ellen K. Chance

The school is a significant factor in intellectual development as well as mental development (Eccles & Roeser, 2011). Adolescents and emerging adults are the largest populations that engage in NSSI behaviors. It is estimated that at least two students in every secondary school classroom engage in NSSI behaviors (Kelada et al., 2017). This makes the impact of school-based approaches a vital component in the treatment of NSSI in children and adolescents. The role of the school counselor as a first responder to mental health issues in schools has implications for both NSSI prevention and intervention. Given the issue of social contagion in children, teen, and young adult populations (White Kress et al., 2004), a tiered prevention approach which considers peer influence in group counseling strategies is critical when addressing NSSI in schools. An interdisciplinary model is presented that includes working with parents, school administration, primary care providers, school counselors, mental health counselors, psychologists, and other youth-serving professionals as a way to efficiently and effectively utilize interdisciplinary approaches in school. Available outcomes-based treatment approaches and prevention and intervention methods are detailed for those working in primary and secondary educational settings.

Role of the school counselor

School counselors often serve as the first access point for school-based mental health services and are the ones to address NSSI through prevention, assessment, intervention, and referral processes. The school counselor, in partnership with other educators, parents/guardians, and the community, seeks to provide services that prevent and respond to NSSI behaviors through the delivery of a comprehensive school counseling program. The American School Counselor Association National Model (ASCA, 2012) provides a framework for comprehensive school counseling that is preventative in design, data-driven and developmental in nature, and where 80% of counselor time is spent providing direct and indirect counseling services to students. According to the ASCA's (2017) position statement, "The Professional School Counselor and the Identification, Prevention and Intervention of Behaviors That Are Harmful and Place Students At-Risk," school counselors are school-based leaders who identify, prevent, and address self-injurious behaviors and are obligated to help students access the resources they need to be successful and resilient. Through both direct and indirect counseling services, school counselors are able to work preventatively while also responding to students who self-injure. Beyond direct services and intervention, school counselors play a critical role in the training and education of school staff, parents, and other key stakeholders in identifying and responding to NSSI, developing school-wide policies that address NSSI, and working toward early identification and intervention for students. Finally, school counselors can be influential in engaging parents/guardians and connecting students and families to mental health services by providing appropriate referrals.

Challenges in schools

The primary challenge that exists in schools is that there are often too few school counselors to handle the many mental health needs of the school. ASCA (2012) recommends a student-to-school-counselor ratio of 250:1, but the average ratio is reported at 471:1. This leaves a large burden for teachers and other staff members. Teachers and other staff need to have some training in identifying mental health issues and, more specifically, the common ones such as bullying, NSSI, dating violence, depression, and anxiety. This is coupled with the responsibility of providing education and a structured learning environment; this added duty is a lot for any teacher, counselor, or staff member to take on. Therefore, self-injury is often ignored, such as in the "Case of Sam;" missed or overlooked, as in the "Case of Jenny;" or assessed incorrectly, as in the "Case of Rick." If your school does not have a protocol, some tips for handling NSSI can be found in Table 9.1, but a protocol should be established. All teachers, assistants, staff, administrators, janitors, coaches, and more need to be trained in self-injury protocol. Due to social contagion, students should not be included in this training, unless they are at risk for NSSI and have been flagged by a school counselor.

Social contagion is the other large problem that exists in school systems. This is when behaviors like NSSI spread in groups, but in a way that is sometimes described as "hypnotic" where people truly believe that they find relief or enjoy that activity. This is different than copycatting and doing something just because your friend or a celebrity does it, and you are trying to fit in. Schools are perfect examples of systems where social contagion can easily happen. During some developmental stages, certain age groups can be more susceptible to social contagion than others. Social contagion occurs due to being around peers who are engaging in NSSI (most often successfully) but it can also happen from watching it being glamorized on television or on the internet, or by having family members who have a history of NSSI. Preventing social contagion can be difficult. That is why having specific NSSI groups in schools is not recommended, whereas holding groups that teach kids and teens social and emotional regulation, distress tolerance, or positive coping skills are just as effective and do not potentially add to social contagion. Additionally, it is

Table 9.1 Do and don't tip sheet for NSSI in schools

General policies for consideration	
DO make yourself aware of policies, laws, and guidelines in addressing NSSI and suicidal ideations in schools.	**DON'T** develop policies without considering local context, nature of the setting, and informed evidence-based approaches.
DO develop a protocol that is specific to NSSI.	**DON'T** combine NSSI and suicide policies into one. They are separate, and one does not equate to the other.
DO develop policies and strategies for things like field trips, bus rides, and after-school activities.	**DON'T** develop a one-size-fits-all policy in regard to these things. Banning students from extracurricular activities and school events could impede treatment.
DO communicate in a way that is calm and supportive.	**DON'T** overreact and get upset or lecture the student.
DO refer to a counselor on staff or other health professional for assistance.	**DON'T** punish the student or send them to deans, principals, or detention for NSSI.
DO use the appropriate language that matches the student's language when addressing it.	**DON'T** talk over students or refer to the self-injury as suicide.
DO educate students in a broad, health-related context.	**DON'T** provide school-based assemblies, newsletters, or other mass ways to address "outbreaks."
DO seek support and guidance from school counselors before calling parents.	**DON'T** automatically call parents and assume that you are helping by doing so.
DO make sure each student engaging in NSSI has a unique and supportive plan in place that includes teachers and support staff.	**DON'T** refer the student out and not address the matter again in school and assume it is not a school-based issue.
DO talk with the student about contagion and why it is important to have a safe place for them to talk about self-injury in a way that is helpful for them, but also that will not affect others.	**DON'T** ignore any student's displaying of injuries and having the conversation about NSSI and contagion.

recommended to ask those who engage in NSSI to avoid sharing specific details with other students, glamorizing the injuries, or visibly displaying wounds and scars from self-injury unnecessarily.

Key elements in protocols

There are several school protocols that exist to help schools work with children and young adults who engage in NSSI. Choosing the right protocol for you and your school is critical to assisting those engaging in NSSI. The protocol will be the guide that all school staff and personnel follow to assist those engaging in NSSI. At a minimum, this will help those who are not trained so that they may identify students who are actively engaging in NSSI and/or share about and refer them to the appropriate channels in the school. This protocol also assists staff who may be uncomfortable handling issues such as NSSI. It takes the questions out of the ways to handle self-injury and allows the student to be assessed and supported faster, which is safer for the student. It is also important to note that protocols for NSSI have overlapping features with protocols for handling suicidal ideation, but they are ultimately different, and one cannot substitute for another. Berger et al. (2015) empirically evaluated all of the elements that are considered essential in school protocols and came up with the following key actions: (a) define the roles and responsibilities of the staff members for responding to the NSSI, which also include training tailored to the various personnel; (b) complete a risk assessment for the student who is self-injuring and determine the risk present; (c) issue referrals as needed after the risk assessment is complete; (d) notify the parent while adhering to the ethical and legal guidelines; and (e) manage social contagion within the school.

Protocols available

Stargell et al. (2017) presented a school counseling protocol, or a fixed course of action, for addressing student self-injury. A strong emphasis should be placed on the importance of establishing and implementing NSSI protocols to ensure student safety and well-being, while remaining within the scope of a school counselor's role and practice. The protocol recommends that staff members should be knowledgeable about the referral process and how to contact a designated mental health professional (DMHP) (e.g., the school counselor) when concern for student self-injury is present. Upon referral, the DMHP would conduct and document a self-injury assessment within one hour of the report to assess for low or high severity. According to Whitlock et al. (2008), high-severity self-injury may be characterized by chronic self-injury, greater tissue damage, multiple means of harming oneself, elevated risk of abuse, and higher risk for suicidality. Stargell et al. (2017) recommends assessing severity based off of the following criteria: "(a) preferred methods for self-injury, (b) frequency of self-injury, (c) depth and severity of wounds, (d) triggers for self-injury, (e) antecedents and consequential results, and (f) wound care" (p. 40). It is important to note that assessment of physical injuries should be conducted by a school-based medical professional and is outside the scope of practice for school counselors (Stargall et al., 2017). As recommended next steps, the authors assert that an initial suicide risk assessment should be conducted regardless of high or low severity of self-injury. The use of standardized assessment is encouraged, as results of such measures can be considered more reliable and valid. Examples of such scales include the Columbia Suicide Severity Rating Scale (C-SSRS; Posner et al., 2011), the Self-Injurious Thoughts and Behaviors

Interview (Nock Holmberg et al., 2013), and the Suicide Attempt Self-Injury Interview (SASII; Linehan et al., 2006). An ongoing suicide risk assessment will be necessary when working with students who self-injure, even if the self-injury is first presented as non-suicidal in nature. The next critical step of the protocol is consultation regarding the school counselor's intended plan of action, to ensure considerations regarding safety, confidentiality, and appropriate referrals are contemplated. Before creating a personalized student safety plan, the parents of the student and the supervisor/principal of the school counselor should be apprised and brought in for collaboration. According to Stargall et al. (2017), the safety plan serves as documentation of the NSSI protocol and, most importantly, facilitates student safety and wellness. Finally, as previously stated, it is essential for school counselors to work within their personal scope of practice (ASCA, 2016); thus, an essential component of a school counselor's response to NSSI is to provide referrals to outside mental health professionals to the students involved in self-injurious behaviors and to their parents/guardians.

Cornell's self-injury protocol

Cornell Research Program on Self-Injury and Recovery (Bubrick et al., 2010) has developed a school protocol for responding to NSSI in schools utilizing evidence-based best practices. The protocol was created for school staff and faculty, specifically counselors, nurses, administrators, and other support personnel, and provides a clear process for detecting and responding to self-injury in the school setting. The functional school protocol includes clear steps and a useful flowchart for following a standardized process. According to Bubrick et al. (2010), a school counselor should adhere to the following steps:

1. *Identify self-injury*: injury can be reported through student disclosure, peer disclosure, or when teacher/staff or another adult notices warning signs and symptoms.
2. *Assess self-injury*: note the severity (i.e., superficial, battery/light tissue damage, or chronic/high severity), frequency, and function of the self-injury, as well as risk for suicide. Bubrick et al. (2010) state, "Overall, questions should aim to assess (a) history, (b) frequency, (c) types of methods used, (d) triggers, (e) psychological purpose, (f) disclosure, (g) help-seeking and support, and (h) history and current presence of suicidal ideation and/or behavior" (p. 5).
3. *Designate individuals to serve as the point person at the school*: a designated staff member (e.g., counselor, psychologist, social worker) manages next steps, including parental notification/involvement, school-based intervention and management, and external referral sources.
4. *Determine under what circumstances parents should be contacted*: driven by state and local laws regarding confidentiality and parent disclosure, each school must create its protocol for engaging parents in adherence to these regulations.

5. *Manage active student self-injury (with the self-injurious student, peers, parents, and external referrals)*: for low-risk cases, the point person will provide counseling services geared toward building healthy coping skills and creating a safety and follow up plan. For moderate to high-risk cases, the point person will inform the parent and student of the process for seeking external services and make appropriate referrals.
6. *Determine when and how to issue an outside referral*: moderate to high-risk cases should be referred to external providers, ideally those who specialize and have training in self-injury. This often requires the point person to work closely with the family to inform about services and encourage treatment.
7. *Identify external referral sources and contact information*: Bubrick et al. (2010) recommend utilizing sources such as the S.A.F.E. Alternatives website (selfinjury.com/referrals) to find clinicians who specialize in self-injury. Other recommendations include searching both the state and local counseling association website for referral sources and researching agencies and practices within the community.
8. *Educate staff and students about self-injury*: a critical element of the protocol is the explicit education and training of all staff members on the signs and symptoms of self-injury, what self-injury is and what is not (i.e., piercings, tattoos, etc.), and the difference between NSSI and suicidal ideation and behaviors. Furthermore, the entire school staff should possess a strong understanding of the NSSI protocol and know the identified point person for addressing NSSI on the school campus.

The case of Sam

The use of this protocol will be applied and highlighted using the "Case of Sam" as an example.

After a teacher begins to recognize that 11-year-old Sam's skin picking has increased in frequency and become a distraction in class, she feels it is best to follow the self-injury protocol she was recently trained on by the school counselor, Ms. Smith, and puts in an immediate referral for counseling. Within an hour of receiving the referral, Ms. Smith holds a session with Sam to assess the severity of the self-injury. Ms. Smith begins the session by building rapport with Sam and demonstrating unconditional regard, reviewing confidentiality and informed consent, and explaining that his teachers were concerned about his well-being. Ms. Smith spends some time exploring the student's experiences with NSSI and the contributing factors and the function of the self-injury. Sam discloses that over the last year, he has been a victim of harsh treatment and bullying by a group of his peers, which has produced strong feelings of anger and disdain toward his peers. He also expressed feelings of loneliness, boredom, and, at times, isolation within his home environment. Sam was able to identify that these strong negative emotions have contributed to his engagement in picking his skin. Ms. Smith provides psychoeducation on NSSI and then conducts a self-injury and suicide risk assessment.

Additionally, Ms. Smith collaborates with the school nurse, who provides a physical evaluation of Sam's wounds. At this time, Sam's wounds are not life-threatening or infected; however, the nurse discusses the physical and safety concerns related to NSSI. Ms. Smith's evaluation concludes low risk for suicide, as Sam did not disclose ideation, intent, or plan for a suicide attempt. However, the assessment does inform Ms. Smith that Sam is at high risk of continued NSSI, as he was assessed at the chronic/high severity level. At this point, Ms. Smith reminds Sam of her responsibility to his safety and well-being and discusses with Sam how to involve his mother in creating a safety plan (see Appendix B). She consults with the contract school mental health counselor to discuss her plan of action. Sam's mother is called by both Ms. Smith and Sam and comes to the school to be involved in the safety planning process. Together, they discuss specific health strategies for coping with negative emotions and his reported feelings of isolation, establish a safety plan for home, create a detailed strategy for open communication, and generate a student support contact list at school. Ms. Smith discusses community-based mental health services and provides Sam's mother with a list of referrals. Finally, feedback is submitted to the administration and referring staff within the confines of confidentiality.

In addition to having a standardized protocol for responding to NSSI, counselors should work proactively to promote protective factors for NSSI. By utilizing a tiered approach within the comprehensive school counseling framework, school counselors can be impactful in addressing NSSI at three levels: (1) primary prevention, (2) secondary prevention, and (3) tertiary care (Wester et al., 2017). This tiered approach will be discussed in depth in the next section.

Tiered response to intervention for NSSI in schools

Creating and sustaining a comprehensive framework for addressing NSSI within the school setting is necessary for both prevention and early intervention. Utilizing a multi-tiered counseling framework, a range of school-wide practices and interventions can be implemented on a continuum to address the needs of students effectively (ASCA, 2014). Moreover, the framework works to ensure that all students are reached and that the appropriate intensity of school-based services is provided. The tiered process is data-driven and ranges from primary prevention/universal prevention to secondary intervention to intensive intervention.

Tier 1: Primary prevention

Tier 1 supports are implemented school-wide as preventative services, and also for early identification and intervention. Various preventative approaches should be implemented at this level, including the promotion of social-emotional competence, emotional regulation and stress reduction, and social connectedness, as well as increased knowledge of NSSI for both students and school personnel. In tiered approaches, is anticipated that approximately 80% of students' needs will be met through Tier 1 supports and interventions (Wells & Axe, 2013).

According to the Cornell Research Program on Self-Injury and Recovery (Bubrick et al., 2010), promoting social connectedness, emotional regulation, and coping skills is effective in the prevention of NSSI. Thus, Tier 1 primary prevention for NSSI within schools should work to promote the social-emotional skills and competence of students; provide learning opportunities for how to cope with adversity and negative emotions; and create a safe, encouraging school climate that encourages connectedness. The goal of Tier 1 intervention is to promote the development of healthy and socially and emotionally competent students who possess the ability to cope with negative emotions. Many school-wide efforts can be implemented to reach this goal, such as direct instruction and promotion of social-emotional learning, and mental health awareness and prevention efforts. Early intervention and prevention, in the form of an explicit social-emotional learning (SEL) curriculum, is vital to the development of social-emotional competence and skill development, and ultimately the life outcomes of students (White & Kelly, 2010).) When school-based SEL programs are well designed and well implemented, they create significant positive impacts across a broad range of student outcomes, including positive effects on student well-being and mental health (Durlak et al., 2011). A significant impact of SEL in schools is the increased ability for students to recognize and manage their emotions, particularly the regulation of negative emotions (Denham, 2006). Emotion regulation is often a function of self-injury (Stargell et al., 2017); thus, equipping students, preventatively, to cope with negative emotions and enhance their self-regulation can ultimately serve as a protective factor for NSSI. The Collaborative for Academic, Social and Emotional Learning (CASEL, 2012) program guides can be useful to schools in identifying and selecting efficacious SEL programs. CASEL (2012) utilizes a systematic framework for identifying, evaluating, and rating SEL programs, and shares best-practice guidelines for schools and districts.

In addition to primary prevention efforts, for early intervention for NSSI, school staff and students must be equipped to identify signs of NSSI and students in distress (Lieberman et al., 2009). Furthermore, they must be informed of a process for seeking assistance within the school if self-harm or student distress is suspected. While peers are often the first to know (Evans et al., 2005), they may be unlikely to report if they have not been oriented on how to respond and report. Thus, a critical element of early intervention is having a distinct process for reporting concerns for student safety and well-being. Berger et al. (2015) assert that appropriate management of NSSI in schools requires clear and well-communicated response protocols. Additionally, above and beyond clear communication is also the importance of creating a safe, welcoming, trusting and encouraging environment in which students feel connected and more apt to trust the process of reporting.

The case of Charlotte

Charlotte has had a history of NSSI since the age of 15. She has many risk factors for NSSI, which include abuse, a history of depression, and identifying as bisexual. Her mother intervened before Charlotte went to college, and she was engaged in therapy and able to stop self-injuring for a period of time, which is a protective factor. Now that Charlotte is in college, primary intervention on college campuses can help prevent some of what she is currently experiencing. Charlotte is willing to engage in therapy, which likely means she may have continued some form of therapy or groups upon entering college. These groups could have assisted her with emotional regulation and stress reduction. The transition from home to college and the new academic and life pressures were likely too much for Charlotte to cope with. This transition period can be critical for an adolescent. She is in a new place and expected to make new friends. She is also not out to her family regarding her sexual orientation, and she has a new girlfriend. Talking with a therapist about this could help, but more social connectedness with others in similar situations can be achieved in primary prevention efforts on campus. She could have connected with others who identify as LGBTQI+ or those who self-injure in support groups. Connecting with others who are similar is important for her development, but also her social and emotional well-being. Campus-wide efforts could have been implemented, including mental health awareness and prevention efforts. This could have helped Charlotte not to feel stigmatized. Additionally, educational programs and groups to support healthy eating patterns and healthy lifestyle choices could assist her in decision-making about restricting food intake. Even though Charlotte is on her own and in college, she never shared her struggles and her NSSI history or her gender and affectional orientation with her parents. As she enters college and is now on her own and independent, she will start to form her identity, but also new intimate relationships fully. Since she was cooperative with therapy in the past and was able to stop engaging in NSSI before she went to college, it is likely she would be willing to engage in some of these preventative measures once she reached college.

At all levels of the multi-tiered framework, it is critical to utilize efficacious, evidence-based approaches for addressing NSSI. At the Tier 1 level, consideration of an evidence-based prevention program for students and professional learning for staff is recommended. While the evaluation of school-based NSSI prevention programs is limited, promising research has been conducted on The Signs of Self-Injury program developed by Screening for Mental Health, Inc. (SOSI, Jacobs et al., 2009; Muehlenkamp, Walsh, & McDade, 2010; Walsh & Muehlenkamp, 2013). This comprehensive prevention program offers a psychoeducational training for school personnel, and also offers one module for students to learn about the signs and symptoms of NSSI and how to appropriately respond when peers, or self, engage in NSSI. According to Muehelenkamp et al. (2010), the goals of the SOSI program are to: "(a) increase knowledge of NSSI including warning signs and symptoms, (b) improve attitudes and perceived capability to respond and help refer students, or peers, who engage in NSSI, (c) increase help-seeking behaviors for NSSI for peers or self, and (d) decrease acts of NSSI among adolescents" (p. 307). Results from the study conducted by Muehelenkamp et al. (2010) suggest that the SOSI school-based program is effective in adolescent self-reported increased knowledge of NSSI, openness to seek help for peers or self, and decreased discomfort with and avoidance of NSSI in friends. Equally important, the study found that the SOSI program did not have iatrogenic effects or self-injury contagion.

Tier 2: Secondary prevention

Tier 2 supports are intended for students whose needs are not met by Tier 1 interventions. Through targeted small group and individualized interventions, emerging or low-risk NSSI and mental health needs can be addressed. Tier 2 interventions should be developed utilizing data-driven practices and should be targeted and unique to each student. The goal of Tier 2 is to reduce or eliminate self-injurious behaviors or mental health concerns while building social-emotional competence for healthier functioning. School-based targeted interventions are usually short term (approximately 6–16 weeks). It is anticipated that 15% of the student population will need Tier 2 intervention (Wells & Axe, 2013).

Small group counseling interventions

Research on the effectiveness of group interventions for addressing NSSI presents important considerations for all mental health professionals, including the risk of social contagion (Richardson et al., 2012; Walsh, 2006). While the benefits of group intervention includes decreasing feelings of isolation, increasing student connectedness, and universalizing, researchers suggest that the potential for social contagion is significant (Richardson et al., 2012; Walsh, 2006). With this in mind, school-based counselors and mental health professionals should be strategic when forming and facilitating groups for students engaging in NSSI. It should be done with extreme caution due to social contagion. One consideration is to group students who engage in NSSI with students who do not, but who are all in need of learning coping skills, mindfulness, stress management, and so on. This promotes balance within the group and removes the criterion for participation and focus from self-injury itself. According to Richardson et al. (2012), if groups are formed for only students who engage in NSSI, there should be a very specific structure and clear guidelines communicated to participants. First, group leaders should have a high level of training and understanding of treating NSSI and managing social contagion. Second, to promote social cohesion and trust, closed membership is advised. Third, the group should set a strict guideline to prohibit discussion of NSSI and wound/scar sharing, and all members should commit to abiding by this guideline for participation in the group. Finally, the group should be highly structured and focus on promoting emotional regulation, coping skills, social-emotional skills, and competence.

The case of Rick

In light of Rick's father refusing a referral for external services, the psychologist puts a referral in for school-based counseling services. The school counselor determines that Rick has a moderate severity of self-injurious behavior and would greatly benefit from small-group counseling services that focus on promoting self-regulation, positive coping skills, and enhancing social-emotional competence. The father consents to school counseling services, and Rick begins participation in an eight-week, closed group with five other students who have a variety of presenting concerns, not exclusively students who self-harm. Through participating in the group, Rick becomes less angry and volatile over situations and can use some of his learned coping skills on occasion, which in turn decreases the number of physical fights he engages in at school. Additionally, Rick is provided some tangible tools and skills that he can utilize individually outside of groups to help gauge his anger (see Appendix J).

Tier 2: Individualized interventions

Students engaging in NSSI are certain to need varying levels of individualized intervention. Within schools, individualized interventions are likely to be provided by the school counselor, school-based or school contracted mental health counselor, and/or school psychologist or school social worker. According to Shapiro et al. (2013), evidence-based treatment approaches for adolescent NSSI can be feasible within the school setting, and there is some evidence pointing to the effectiveness of cognitive-behavioral therapy, dialectical behavior therapy, and problem-solving therapy interventions, as discussed in the previous chapter.

A manualized cognitive-behavioral therapy intervention, Cutting Down (Taylor et al., 2011), has demonstrated effectiveness in addressing NSSI, specifically self-cutting. The 14-session program provides psychoeducation, teaches effective coping strategies, identifies cognitive distortions, and promotes relapse prevention. An evaluation of the program found that student participation resulted in reduced NSSI, and a reduction in both depression and anxiety symptoms, which was maintained by three months post-treatment (Taylor et al., 2011).

Tier 3: Tertiary care

Tier 3 supports are enacted for students with more severe or chronic NSSI. A multi-disciplinary team referral results in individual therapeutic intervention provided by the appropriate school-based mental health professional, and a referral is made to an outside community mental health provider. School-wide crisis response protocols are enacted when necessary in addressing severe cases of NSSI. The overall goal of the Tier 3 level of support is to connect the student and families to the appropriate professionals for addressing NSSI and can include referral to intensive outpatient or inpatient programs. At this level, school counseling professionals function as the liaison between students, families, and treatment facilities. In addition, they facilitate student reentry to school following hospitalizations, or inpatient treatment services, and can serve as a check-in for students.

The case of Emma

With the understanding that Emma's NSSI has been chronic and severe, coupled with symptoms of suicidal ideation and hospitalizations, the school counselor assumes the role of liaison between the treatment facility and the school. The school counselor seeks consent for a release of information with the hospital from the guardian. Upon consent, the counselor obtains discharge records that include information on medication, treatment, and safety planning and recommendations for the school setting. The counselor works with the family to ensure safety plans are in place at the school and establishes daily check-ins with Emma for the foreseeable future. Finally, the counselor frequently follows up with the guardian and external provider to monitor student well-being and progress in therapy.

Summary

Utilizing an interdisciplinary, tiered prevention and intervention approach to addressing NSSI in primary and secondary educational settings, counseling professionals can work to prevent, reduce, and eliminate self-injurious behaviors. Furthermore, by applying the appropriate evidence-based prevention and intervention approaches, counselors can help students cope with stressors and negative emotions in adaptive rather than self-defeating ways, while also mitigating the concern for social contagion. The counseling process in school is often made more complex by the function and severity of the NSSI. Thus, the awareness of a clear and well-communicated process and protocol for assessing severity and level of risk, and the knowledge of a range of community resources available, can aide counselors in delivering the most appropriate comprehensive services for students.

REFERENCES

American School Counselor Association. (2012). *The ASCA National Model: A Framework for School Counseling Programs* (3rd ed.). Alexandria, VA: Author. doi:10.1037/e504812012-001

American School Counselor Association. (2014). The school counselor and multitiered systems of support. ASCA *position statements*. Retrieved from http://www.schoolcounselor.org/asca/media/asca/positionstatements/PS_MultitieredSupportSystem.pdf

American School Counselor Association. (2016). *Ethical Standards for School Counselors*. Alexandria, VA: Author.

American School Counselor Association. (2017). The professional school counselor and the identification, prevention and intervention of behaviors that are harmful and place students at-risk ASCA position statements. ASCA *position statements*. Retrieved from https://www.schoolcounselor.org/asca/media/asca/PositionStatements/PositionStatements.pd

Berger, E., Hasking, P., & Reupert, A. (2015). Developing a policy to address nonsuicidal self-injury in schools. *Journal of School Health*, 85(9), 629–647. doi:10.1111/josh.12292

Bubrick, K., Goodman, J., & Whitlock, J. (2010). Non-suicidal self-injury in schools: Developing and implementing school protocol. [Fact sheet] Cornell Research Program on Self-Injurious Behavior in Adolescents and Young Adults. Retrieved from http://www.selfinjury.bctr.cornell.edu/documents/schools.pdf

Collaborative for Academic, Social, and Emotional Learning. (2012). *2013 CASEL Guide: Effective Social and Emotional Learning Programs—Preschool and Elementary School Edition*. Chicago, IL: Author. Retrieved from https://casel.org/preschool-and-elementary-edition-casel-guide/

Denham, S.A. (2006). Social-emotional competence as support for school readiness: What is it and how do we assess it? *Early Education & Development*, 17(1), 57–89. doi:10.1207/s15566935eed1701_4

Durlak, J.A., Weissberg, R.P., Dymnicki, A.B., Taylor, R.D., & Schellinger, K.B. (2011). The impact of enhancing students' social and emotional learning: A meta-analysis of school-based universal interventions. *Child Development*, 82(1), 405–432. doi:10.1111/j.1467-8624.2010.01564.x

Eccles, J.S., & Roeser, R.W. (2011). Schools as developmental contexts during adolescence. *Journal of Research on Adolescence*, 21(1), 225–241. doi:10.1111/j.1532-7795.2010.00725.x

Evans, E., Hawton, K., & Rodham, K. (2005). In what ways are adolescents who engage in self-harm or experience thoughts of self-harm different in terms of help-seeking, communication and coping strategies? *Journal of Adolescence*, 28, 573–587. doi:10.1016/j.adolescence.2004.11.001

Jacobs, D., Walsh, B.W., McDade, M., & Pigeon, S. (2009). *Signs of Self-Injury Prevention Manual*. Wellesley Hills, MA: Screening for Mental Health.

Kelada, L., Hasking, P., & Melvin, G.A. (2017). School response to self-injury: Concerns of mental health staff and parents. *School Psychology Quarterly*, 32(2), 173–187. doi:10.1037/spq0000194

Lieberman, R.A., Toste, J.R., & Heath, N.L. (2009). Nonsuicidal self-injury in the schools: Prevention and intervention. In: M.K. Nixon & N.L. Heath (Eds.), *Self-Injury in Youth: The Essential Guide to Assessment and Intervention* (pp. 195–216). New York, NY: Taylor & Francis. doi:10.4324/9780203892671

Linehan, M.M., Comtois, K.A., Brown, M.Z., Heard, H.L., & Wagner, A. (2006). Suicide Attempt Self-Injury Interview (SASII): Development, reliability, and validity of a scale to assess suicide attempts and intentional self-injury. *Psychological Assessment*, 18(3), 303–312. doi:10.1037/1040-3590.18.3.303

Muehlenkamp, J.J., Walsh, B.W., & McDade, M. (2010). Preventing non-suicidal self-injury in adolescents: The signs of self-injury program. *Journal of Youth & Adolescence*, 39, 306–314. doi:10.1007/s10964-009-9450-8

Nock, M.K., Holmberg, E.B., Photos, V.I., Michel, B.D., Shingleton, R.M., Eddy, K.T., & Herzog, D.B. (2013). Self-Injurious Thoughts and Behaviors Interview. *International Journal of Eating Disorders*, 46(7), 684–689.

Posner, K., Brown, G.K., Stanley, B., Brent, D.A., Yershova, K.V., Oquendo, M.A., … Mann, J.J. (2011). The Columbia-Suicide Severity Rating Scale: Initial validity and internal consistency findings from three multisite studies with adolescents and adults. *American Journal of Psychiatry*, 168(12), 1266–1277. doi:10.1176/appi.ajp.2011.10111704

Richardson, B.G., Surmitis, K.A., & Hyldahl, R.S. (2012). Minimizing social contagion in adolescents who self-injure: Considerations for group work, residential treatment, and the internet. *Journal of Mental Health Counseling*, 34(2), 121. doi:10.17744/mehc.34.2.206j243468882617

Shapiro, A., Heath, N., & Roberts, E. (2013). Treatment of nonsuicidal self-injury: Critical review and implications for school applications. *School Psychology Forum*, 7(4), 121.

Stargell, N.A., Zoldan, C.A., Kress, V.E., Walker-Andrews, L.M., & Whisenhunt, J.L. (2017). Student non-suicidal self-injury: A protocol for school counselors. *Professional School Counseling*, 21(1). doi:10.5330/1096-2409-21.1.37

Taylor, L.M.W., Oldershaw, A., Richards, C., & Davidson, K. (2011). Development and pilot evaluation of a manualized cognitive-behavioral treatment package for adolescent self-harm. *Behavioural and Cognitive Psychotherapy*, 39(5), 619–625. doi:10.1017/s1352465811000075

Walsh, B. (2006). *Treating Self-Injury: A Practical Guide*. New York, NY: Guilford Press.

Walsh, B., & Muehlenkamp, J.J. (2013). Managing nonsuicidal self-injury in schools: Use of a structured protocol to manage the behavior and prevent social contagion. *School Psychology Forum*, 7(4), 161–171. Retrieved from http://www.nasponline.org/

Wells, A., & Axe, J.B. (2013). A three-tiered approach for addressing nonsuicidal self-injury in the classroom. *Beyond Behavior*, 22(2), 35. doi:10.1177/107429561302200207

Wester, K.L., Morris, C.W., & Williams, B. (2017). Nonsuicidal self-injury in the schools: A tiered prevention approach for reducing social contagion. *Professional School Counseling*, 21(1). doi:10.5330/1096-2409-21.1.142

White, S.W., & Kelly, F.D. (2010). The school counselor's role in school dropout prevention. *Journal of Counseling & Development*, 88(2), 227–235. doi:10.1002/j.1556-6678.2010.tb00014.x

White Kress, V.E., Gibson, D.M., & Reynolds, C.A. (2004). Adolescents who self-injure: Implications and strategies for school counselors. *Professional School Counseling*, 7, 195–201.

Whitlock, J., Muehlenkamp, J., & Eckenrode, J. (2008). Variation in nonsuicidal self-injury: Identification and features of latent classes in a college population of emerging adults. *Journal of Clinical Child & Adolescent Psychology*, 37(4), 725–735. doi:10.1080/15374410802359734

10 Treatment in community settings

Adriana Labarta and Bridget Glass

In various community settings, professional counselors will likely encounter clients who engage in NSSI. Therefore, it is crucial to become familiar with effective treatment strategies that can be utilized and adapted for diverse clients. A counselor's theoretical orientation can certainly influence how they approach treatment. For example, a narrative counselor may encourage clients to externalize the NSSI, which helps shift client perspective to empowerment and autonomy and away from feelings of shame. Family therapists may address communication issues that have caused ruptures within the client's family system to promote supportive engagement among its members. Those conceptualizing clients from a feminist perspective may consider the impact of societal influence, gender issues, and cultural oppression while empowering clients to reclaim autonomy and create sustainable change for themselves and those around them struggling with similar life issues.

Due to the clinical severity and prevalence of NSSI in mental health and community settings, criteria from the American Psychological Association Task Force assert that no one current treatment for NSSI qualifies as fully empirically-supported, efficacious, or well established (APA, 2002). This is a result of ethical constraints of research with vulnerable populations, such as those who engage in self-injurious behaviors. The current evidence-based, or evidence-supported treatments, and interventions have variable strengths that have been determined from meta-analyses and expert opinions. The specific challenge of evidence-based practices lies in the application of an ethical framework that protects the participant's needs and rights while addressing the researcher's goals and limitations when studying NSSI (Singhal & Bhola, 2017). Nock (2010) notes that there are no treatments for NSSI that could be considered "evidence-based." Despite these challenges, several treatment strategies have emerged wherein researchers indicate efficacious and outcomes-based data with individuals who engage in NSSI. In this chapter, four evidence-based theories that are outcome based for NSSI will be detailed and applied to client cases: eye movement desensitization and reprocessing, family therapy, dialectical behavioral therapy, and cognitive behavioral therapy.

Basic interventions

Counselors must consider three critical keys when treating clients who self-harm: the history of NSSI, developmental stage, and diversity factors. These elements serve to inform clinical treatment and help the counselor select appropriate interventions for an integrative approach. Treatment settings may also affect the suitability of therapeutic intervention. Factors such as duration of treatment and level of structure and support can increase or decrease the potential for successful outcomes. Regardless of what theoretical model is implemented in treatment, it is important to be aware of general interventions that may help facilitate client change. Firstly, the counselor should treat the client with empathy and respect to create a therapeutic environment conducive to openness and growth. Also, the provision of psychoeducation and practice of skills related to communication and assertiveness may enable clients to better advocate for their needs when experiencing urges to self-injure.

Safety planning is an essential intervention for all clients who engage in NSSI. Safety plans should be created collaboratively to identify warning signs, coping strategies, social supports, community resources, and ways to limit access to means that the client may use to self-injure. It is imperative that families be involved in this process when working with child and adolescent populations. Along a similar line is holistic harm reduction models of treatment for adults. The main focus of the treatment and intervention is to seek understanding of the self-injury and the function, in order to provide education to reduce the risks that come with NSSI engagement. NSSI is a problematic coping skill, but providing education on the process helps clients to better be able to express themselves. Ghafoor (2008) offered a controversial intervention in harm reduction by taking education a step further and informing clients on how many cuts to make and how deep to make them. Pembroke (2006) educated clients on anatomy and physiology of the skin to reduce medical intervention and scarring. It was called "supervised harm" and does not condone the self-injury, but instead reduces inherent risk and allows the clients to think before they act and engage in the self-injury process. These are often viewed as last options when all other treatments have been exhausted.

Self-soothing strategies are also useful for clients to help replace NSSI behaviors in treatment. Activities may include journaling, listening to music, deep breathing, being outdoors, or talking to a friend. In a study exploring how self-injurers resist urges to harm themselves, "doing exercise" and "removing the means/instruments typically used to self-harm from the home" were rated as most helpful (Klonsky & Glenn, 2008). With that said, some self-soothing strategies may be harmful if the client presents with comorbid disorders. For example, a client such as Charlotte, who engages in NSSI and eating-disorder behaviors (restricting), may not benefit from exercise as a self-soothing strategy. This is particularly true for those who are in the weight restoration process and do not have medical clearance by an authorized physician. As we explore evidence-based approaches to treat clients who self-injure, it is important that all models be practiced from a basis of the fundamental principles of counseling, as the establishment of a strong therapeutic alliance is a pivotal aspect for client change. Table 10.1 below lists common approaches for NSSI and how they can be utilized in practice.

Attachment-based family therapy

Attachment-based family therapy (ABFT) is an "interpersonal, process-oriented, trauma-focused approach" that integrates "a clear road map" for the recognition and repair of attachment injuries that have occurred within the context of a family's dynamic (Diamond et al., 2016). This model includes five tasks that each have a specific function in healing damage to attachment bonds as the result of trauma (Diamond et al., 2016). When working with individuals who actively engage in self-injurious behaviors, the focus of treatment is shifted from the client's symptomology to dysfunction that has evolved within the family and has caused disruption in attachment between members (Kissil, 2011). Glenn et al. (2015) completed a random control trial with 66 adolescents (74% African American) and those patients receiving ABFT were found to have significantly greater and faster reductions in SI throughout treatment. Therapists who practice from the ABFT model conceptualize the client's self-injury as a response to problems within the family system, rather than the problem in itself (Kissil, 2011).

The case of Jenny

Jenny has used self-harming behaviors throughout the school-aged stage of her psychosocial development. It appears that Jenny's maladaptive behaviors become more prevalent when she is frustrated by difficult tasks. This phase that relates to industry versus inferiority strongly reflects her feelings of success at both school and home. When Jenny does not think her work is acceptable, or others do not recognize her efforts, she may be triggered to engage in self-injury. Additionally, the onset of Jenny's self-injurious behaviors correlates to her mother's pregnancy with her youngest sibling, as well as difficulties experienced in her parents' marriage. Due to Jenny's trauma history and age when these incidents occurred, it is possible that her attachment style was affected. If Jenny's parents were preoccupied with marital discord and the birth of a new baby, one might presume that their focus was diverted to their interpersonal problems and not on the maintenance of a secure attachment with their eldest daughter. One may also speculate that Jenny, seeking comfort and stability, began to employ maladaptive self-injurious behaviors to cope with the stress that she experienced around her, but was outside of her control.

Jenny presents with several qualities that demonstrate attachment-based family therapy as an appropriate intervention for treatment. Jenny and her parents maintain a positive relationship, and they regularly spend time with her, despite living in separate residences. Although Jenny's parents maintain differing

Table 10.1 Common approaches application

Strategy	*Focus*	*Practice*
Motivational interviewing	Directive and client-centered counseling to elicit behavior by exploring and resolving ambivalence.	Explore the pros and cons of continued NSSI engagement. Gauging the readiness for change and confidence to change with scaling. Supporting the client: "It seems you have been working hard to stop self-injuring, which is different than before. What has given you the strength to do this?"
Adlerian therapy	The focus is on forming a relationship, psychological investigation and disclosure, and reinterpretation/ meaning-making.	You are creating a safe environment for the clients to discuss their NSSI and significant influences: personal history, beliefs, and behavior patterns (see Appendix N) followed by a thorough assessment, insight building, and reorientation, which assists in making positive changes. The therapist can engage the client in "acting as if" or "reflecting as if." "How would you act if you were able to stop injuring? What would it feel like to know that you are able to go through life and not self-injure?"
Emotional regulation group therapy	Exploring NSSI by learning skills to regulate emotions through understanding and acceptance, controlling behavior, and meaning-making (or values-based living).	The clinician will help the client identify meaningfulness in areas of their life. These areas will be reinforced as a rationale not to engage in NSSI. Negative emotions will be addressed throughout therapy and then meaningful activities, people, etc. will be reinforced when addressing negative emotions.
Voice movement therapy	Integrated expressive arts therapy that seeks to reduce emotional distress and increase self-awareness via sound-making, singing, expressive writing, massage, movement, and drama activities.	Emotional distress prior to NSSI is discussed. Clients will learn their triggers that cause distressing emotions and increase self-awareness. Then, expressive activities will be utilized in place of NSSI.
Play therapy	Non-directive, client-centered approach that utilizes toys, games, and sandtray to initiate and facilitate client expression through symbolic play.	The therapist will use tracking, reflection, and enlarging the meaning of non-directive play to help the client communicate thoughts and feelings related to self-injury. Games, art, and sand play can be incorporated into treatment to help individuals recognize cognitive associations between self-harming behaviors and internal struggles they may be experiencing.
Narrative therapy	A collaborative approach between the therapist and the client to identify the problem and separate the problem from the person with a strengths-based approach.	Utilizing externalization, exceptions to the problem, reauthoring, and unique outcomes, the client can begin to use their innate skill set to minimize the current problems and focus on building the strengths they already possess. Finding new and existing purpose and meaning in one's story is imperative. (See Appendices C and M.)

opinions in regard to the severity and resolution of her behaviors, they seem to share an overall concern for her well-being and willingness to collaborate for the benefit of their daughter's health. Additionally, Jenny exhibits a high level of social skills, as she is recognized as a leader in her school, regularly participates in team sports, and engages in a support system. All of the aforementioned protective factors indicate Jenny's resilience and an increased potential for a successful treatment outcome.

Task 1 (one session)

From the beginning of treatment, the therapist will strive to build a strong rapport with both Jenny and her parents. A sense of warmth and empathy must be modeled by the therapist from the very first interaction with the family, to ensure that no members perceive any alliance or judgment within the dynamic. The therapist is able to demonstrate a functional attachment style by exhibiting unconditional positive regard toward each participant in Jenny's treatment. This is critical, as some parents have not experienced this level of acceptance and understanding, and therefore struggle with generating attachment in their own families. As the therapist reflects the qualities that contribute to healthy attachment, he or she is laying the groundwork for Jenny and her parents to build upon within their own family. The initial session is conjoint, and the focus of treatment will be on how trust has been compromised in the family, which has caused a rupture in the attachment between Jenny and her parents, instead of her symptoms (Diamond et al., 2016).

Task 2 (two to four sessions)

The therapist will meet individually with Jenny. Jenny and the therapist will explore difficulties that she has experienced in her life, as well as the feelings associated with those circumstances. Additionally, the therapist will help Jenny create a plan for sharing these thoughts and feelings with her parents. During task two, the therapist will empower Jenny to determine what traumas have occurred in her life that she believes have caused a disruption in attachment with her parents and how she plans to share those past hurts with them in future sessions (Diamond et al., 2016).

Task 3 (two to four sessions)

The therapist will meet with Jenny's parents, both together and separately. The therapist will help each parent examine their own experience of the problems within their family structure and how they have been emotionally affected by those issues. This provides the therapist with several opportunities to validate the feelings expressed by Jenny's parents, which further models elements of attachment building. The therapist will work toward providing Jenny's parents with skills that will contribute toward their overall affect tolerance when they eventually listen to their daughter's concerns. This will ensure Jenny's safety when she eventually discusses difficult thoughts and feelings with them. Engaging Jenny in an activity, such as "building a house," will assist her to identify her supports, values, beliefs, and secrets (see Appendix P). The house can be something to build upon with Jenny and eventually have her share with her parents, in hopes that she can continue to recreate the house throughout therapy, which will show where she is progressing.

Task 4 (one to four sessions)

The emphasis of treatment during this task is reattachment (Kissil, 2011). Sessions will consist of conjoint family therapy interventions based on addressing the family's interpersonal problems that have caused pain within their relationships. Jenny will present the experiences and feelings she identified with the therapist in phase one. Jenny's parents will utilize the strategies they learned in phase one to provide their child with empathy and support. A critical feature of this phase is that Jenny believe it is safe for her to communicate her internal struggles with her parents in order to strengthen their bond as a family. By providing Jenny with genuine understanding, free from defensiveness and judgment, her parents are creating a space for her to trust them when she is distressed. Additionally, by talking to her parents, she provides them with relief from having to anticipate her thoughts and feelings, which can further contribute to the relationship. Furthermore, Jenny's parents will be able to offer her comfort, which in turn will decrease her urge to self-soothe through maladaptive behaviors.

Task 5 (1–10 sessions)

Following task four, the family has repaired disruptions in attachment and is actively working toward functioning from a secure base. However, the family's communication patterns may still be dysfunctional as a result of years of engaging in the same cycles. Therefore, the therapist and the family will continue to practice skills that have been previously taught, as well as examine their progress with these changes in their home (Diamond et al., 2016).

Within the scope of treatment, the therapist must be aware of considerations that may impede treatment outcomes when working with children and adolescents who utilize self-injurious behaviors as a means to cope with their difficulties. This is especially critical in the case of suspected child abuse that is perpetrated by one or both of the participating parents. The therapist must ensure the child's emotional and physical safety in and out of the session. Therefore, screening for abuse should be incorporated in phase one to protect the client from any adverse repercussions that may place him or her in jeopardy. Additionally, the therapist should be monitoring the family's readiness for phase two, and exercise caution when moving from phases prior to appropriate skills-building and preparation. Within phase one, the therapist should help parents reflect on any deficits regarding their attachment styles. The therapist must be cognizant of any residual defensiveness demonstrated by a parent that could inhibit treatment goals during phase two. This is also true for assessing parental empathy and the capacity for tolerating their child's pain. Research in the field of attachment-based family therapy in the treatment of self-injury has been primarily studied with adolescent populations. However, due to factors such as Jenny's maturity and positive indicators for the family's potential for change, it seems that this may be a helpful treatment approach to explore with this family. A final point to consider when working with parents who are divorced, such as in the case of Jenny, is that treatment should include an examination of parental guilt or self-blame resulting from their child's self-injurious behaviors. It is possible that, despite obstacles, some divorced parents can still act as a unit to help their children mend attachment wounds. Individuals who can work together, fostering adaptive emotional regulation in their children and themselves, may discover a new structure within their dynamic and build a unique path toward family healing.

Eye movement desensitization and reprocessing

Eye movement desensitization and reprocessing (EMDR) is an integrative psychotherapy approach that has been extensively researched and proven effective for the treatment of trauma. According to the EMDR International Association (EMDRIA), "EMDR is a set of standardized protocols that incorporate elements from many different treatment approaches" (emdria.org). Within the scope of the approach, clinicians utilize the adaptive information processing (AIP) model as a means "to guide history taking, case conceptualization, treatment planning, and interventions and to predict treatment outcome" (Mosquera & Ross, 2016, p. 119). EMDR practitioners conceptualize non-suicidal self-injurious behavior as a trauma-driven coping strategy utilized by individuals who maintain a limited capacity for self-regulation (Mosquera & Ross, 2016). When treatment outcomes are successful, those who engage in SI can replace previous self-destructive patterns with healthier, more adaptive skills (Mosquera & Ross, 2016). EMDR is a compassionate approach to the treatment of self-injurious behavior, as the practitioner identifies the condition as a response to prior traumatic experiences, as opposed to manipulation or opportunity to seek attention from others (Healey & Craigen, 2010). Unlike other therapeutic approaches, success in treatment is not contingent upon the client verbalizing a detailed account of traumatic events, thus providing additional safety from the risk of further traumatization (Healey & Craigen, 2010). EMDR therapists recognize that those who use self-injury for grounding themselves or to self-sooth do so because it has proven beneficial for them during traumatic or stressful circumstances (Mosquera & Ross, 2016). Factors within the construct of EMDR, such as resource development and installation (RDI), help clients learn effective coping strategies that can then replace previous self-injurious behaviors with those intended to increase long-term stabilization (Mosquera & Ross, 2016). Research for EMDR as an effective treatment model for the prevention of self-injurious behavior is limited. This deficit may be correlated to a shift in perspective from non-suicidal self-injury being the presenting problem to symptomatic of unresolved trauma.

The case of Rhonda

Rhonda is in the psychosocial stage of development of young adulthood. It is possible that her marital discord may have exacerbated an inner conflict, as she once experienced intimacy with her husband but now may be feeling a sense of loneliness and isolation. It is also worthy to note that Rhonda began to engage in self-injurious behaviors during her adolescence. This may have been a time in Rhonda's life when she experienced confusion regarding her identity. The discomfort within herself may have triggered self-harming tactics as a way to self-regulate her overwhelming emotions.

Rhonda demonstrates several protective factors that may indicate her potential for an overall successful outcome following EMDR treatment. Most prominently, Rhonda has been able to terminate self-injurious behaviors for the majority of her adult life. Additionally, Rhonda has actively sought help for her behaviors from both a psychiatrist and a professional counselor, despite high demands at work and home. Moreover, Rhonda has been able to access her support system to help when attending weekly counseling sessions. Finally, Rhonda exhibits a high level of motivation for eliminating cutting behaviors due to her concern regarding judgment from those who may question the state of her mental health and ability to parent. Although this factor may also stimulate her anxious feelings, often precipitating her urge to self-injure, it also demonstrates the level of importance she identifies with healing, which is a critical factor for positive outcomes in the EMDR approach.

Phase 1: Client history & treatment planning

Rhonda's therapist must first determine information that may reveal the impetus of her self-injurious behaviors. In her presentation, Rhonda admits to engaging in self-injury at age 15, yet she provides minimal details regarding this time in her life. At the start of treatment, the therapist should explore the possibility of childhood trauma occurring in Rhonda's history. Traumatic childhood events may have prompted Rhonda to employ cutting herself as a self-soothing strategy. Though maladaptive in nature, these behaviors could have helped Rhonda cope during times of distress (Mosquera & Ross, 2016). The therapist may choose to use the Adverse Childhood Experiences (ACEs) survey to initiate a normative conversation related to Rhonda's past (Shapiro, 2018). This tool may provide the therapist with a further understanding of Rhonda's earliest recollections, as well as indicating any dissociation that may have occurred as a result of trauma (Shapiro, 2018). These factors will be necessary to proceed with the remainder of the EMDR protocol. It is of equal importance for the therapist to examine what caused Rhonda to discontinue self-injury in her early to mid-20s.

Perhaps her marriage or the birth of her children precluded her from the use of self-destructive measures to manage daily stressors. It is interesting to note that Rhonda was able to suspend these behaviors, despite the existence of domestic violence during her marriage. During phase one, it is imperative for the therapist to gather as much information as the client will allow regarding prior trauma. These data points will be used by the therapist in phases three through seven to target memories that are related to the onset of the maladaptive behaviors. Throughout this time, the therapist will aim to dispel negative beliefs that activate Rhonda's urge to self-injure to terminate the behaviors in their entirety (Mosquera & Ross, 2016). Activities that Rhonda can practice at home to reflect on negative beliefs and reframe them will assist in her goal to stop the NSSI (such as in Appendix K).

Phase 2: Preparation

In the preparation phase, the therapist will continue to identify and understand Rhonda's past experiences that may be connected to self-injurious behavior. Rhonda and her therapist will also explore tools that are intended to provide her with emotional safety, as she proceeds throughout the subsequent phases of treatment (Mosquera & Ross, 2016). Resource development and installation is key to preparing the client for processing the target memories. Long term, Rhonda will use learned skills to replace previous cutting behaviors when she experiences distress. Most importantly, the therapist will explain to Rhonda the course of treatment and any risks associated with the approach (Greenwald, 2012).

Phase 3: Assessment

Rhonda and the therapist will determine specific memories that will be targeted during the following phases. For each memory that the therapist will target, Rhonda will be asked to indicate the worst part of the memory and her current Subjective Units Of Distress Scale (SUDS) while reflecting on the memory (Greenwald, 2012). Additionally, Rhonda will explore negative cognitions that she may have as a result of the event she is exploring and a thought that she would prefer to believe instead. This phase is vital, as it informs the therapist about what memories should be processed and the order in which they should be addressed.

Phase 4: Desensitization

The therapist will use eye movements in conjunction with a guided script to engage Rhonda in focusing on targeted memories. Throughout this phase, Rhonda will explore the target memory until she no longer experiences a physical or emotional response upon reflection. The therapist will gauge this change by monitoring Rhonda's body language, her interactions, and fluctuations in her reported SUDS.

Phase 5: Installation

During installation, Rhonda will be challenged to replace previously held negative cognitions with positive beliefs regarding herself or the memory. This is accomplished by utilizing the same process as stated in phase four; however, instead of focusing on the targeted memory, Rhonda will be directed to concentrate on her new, adaptive cognition.

Phase 6: Body scan

The therapist will refocus Rhonda's concentration to the originally targeted memory. Together, they will investigate residual somatic responses that may still be present in her body. The therapist will ask Rhonda to call attention to any sensations she may be experiencing and where those feelings are located. Any report of tension or physical discomfort is an indicator to the therapist that the memory was not fully processed during phases four and five. The therapist will then return to phase four and repeat the steps through phase six until all aspects of the targeted memory have been resolved.

Phase 7: Closure

Within phase seven, the therapist will protect Rhonda's emotional safety by concluding the session with a buffering activity intended to help her regulate her emotions following the protocol. This may be accomplished through a guided imagery exercise for containing troubling thoughts and feelings throughout the week until the next appointment. Closure can also be achieved by engaging in conversation regarding upcoming plans that are unrelated to the target memory. The therapist must allow for the time within the session for closure, as it is necessary to assess the client's mental status before allowing her or him to return to outside responsibilities. The therapist should also help Rhonda create a plan following her first EMDR session. This would occur during the preparation phase and could include items such as not returning to work after the session, reaching out to her support system, rest, and checking in with her therapist that evening.

Phase 8: Reevaluation

Each session, Rhonda and her therapist will briefly review her progress during the week. This will be indicated in a shift in cognition, changes in attitude about self or others, fluctuation in SUDS, and ultimately the completion of self-injurious behaviors. The therapist will use this phase of treatment to re-examine treatment goals and assessment for termination of care.

The therapist must ensure client safety by continually assessing readiness and distress tolerance throughout treatment (Mosquera & Ross, 2016). Throughout phases three through seven, clients may vacillate between the desire to process the traumatic event and not wanting to re-experience it. Additionally, thoughts of suicide or self-injury may increase (Mosquera & Ross, 2016). The therapist must provide the client with this information during the preparation phase, so that appropriate safety planning can be initiated. Additionally, the therapist must use clinical judgment when targeting memories by remaining mindful of the client's SUDS reports during the assessment phase (Mosquera & Ross, 2016).

Dialectical behavioral therapy

Dialectical behavioral therapy was developed by Marsha Linehan (1993) to treat individuals with borderline personality disorder (BPD), of which NSSI is the main symptom. DBT is rooted in cognitive behavioral therapy, Zen Buddhism, problem-solving, and skills-based strategies. Within this framework lies the core dialectic of DBT: the balance of acceptance and change. Since DBT addresses both NSSI and suicidal behaviors, many studies do not differentiate between the two, which are then collectively identified as "parasuicide." Therefore, interpretation of research studies warrants caution (Miller & Smith, 2008; Muehlenkamp, 2006).

DeCou et al. (2019) completed controlled trials that assessed both suicidality and self-directed violence, including NSSI, suicide attempts, suicidal ideation, and accessing psychiatric crisis services. The 18 controlled trails revealed that DBT helped to reduce self-directed violence. In a different study, Stanley et al. (2007) found that brief DBT (DBT-B) produces a significant reduction in NSSI, urges to self-injure, subjective distress, self-rated depression, suicidal ideation, and hopelessness. DBT has also been found to be effective for the adolescent population. Rathus and Miller (2002) developed DBT-A, an adaptation of standard adult DBT, which helped to reduce NSSI by addressing skills deficits among the adolescent population in both individual therapy and family group formats (Mehlum et al., 2014). Cumulative results indicated that DBT contributed to reduced frequency and severity of NSSI suicidal behavior in adolescents (MacPherson et al., 2013).

DBT consists of four core skills and teaching modules: mindfulness, emotion regulation, interpersonal effectiveness, and distress tolerance. Distress tolerance plays a key role in dysregulated behaviors, such as NSSI, as individuals with low distress tolerance are likely to self-injure more frequently (Anestis et al., 2014). In findings from both clinical and non-clinical samples, people who engage in NSSI cease distressing tasks significantly earlier than those who do not self-injure (Gratz et al., 2006; Nock & Mendes, 2008). DBT theorizes that emotion dysregulation is essential to treat since it often leads to impulsive and maladaptive behaviors, including self-injury and inflexible thinking (DeCou et al., 2019).

The case of Charlotte

These factors as mentioned above are present in the case of Charlotte, who is engaging in behaviors that allow her to escape from the emotional discomfort of her childhood sexual trauma and coming-out process, such as NSSI and food restriction. Charlotte's distress can be understood by considering her stage of development in Erikson's developmental theory: identity versus role confusion. For several years of her adolescence, Charlotte struggled with understanding and accepting her sexual identity. She feels fearful of disclosing her new relationship to her family and has turned to NSSI to tolerate her distress with the coming-out process. Although she abstained from engaging in NSSI for six months after previous treatment, it appears that her recent transition from being a high school student to a college student has also contributed to her symptom use. Since Charlotte is limited to six sessions at the university counseling center, DBT will be adapted to meet her needs within a briefer time period. DBT is structured and skills based, which will allow the therapist to address and rotate through the four core skills and teaching modules of DBT.

Session one

The first session should consist of rapport building, psychoeducation, assessment, and safety planning. Due to the brevity of treatment, termination should also be discussed from the very first session. Most importantly, the therapist should aim to create a safe, comfortable space for Charlotte by validating her recent struggles. It is likely that Charlotte completed an initial intake prior to her first session, but the therapist should complete a safety assessment and ask about any recent NSSI. Since Charlotte has a previous treatment history, it may be helpful to ask what was helpful about past counseling that contributed to the termination of NSSI for six months. This self-report feedback will help inform the therapist's approach to best meet the needs of the client. The therapist will then transition into providing psychoeducation on DBT, including the efficacy and structure of treatment. Lastly, time should be dedicated to safety planning to ensure that Charlotte can keep herself safe and resist urges to engage in NSSI. The therapist can introduce the DBT diary card as a tool to self-monitor the agreed-upon target behaviors that occur throughout the week. This will serve as a guide to begin each session and will help Charlotte increase awareness of her daily emotions, urges, and behaviors.

Sessions two to three

The second and third sessions will begin with a review of Charlotte's diary card from the past week. If she engaged in NSSI or another maladaptive behavior since the last session, Charlotte and the therapist would complete a behavioral chain analysis of the target behavior (see Appendix G), describing the moment-to-moment chain of events, antecedents, and consequences of the target behavior. The therapist should model the use of dialectics through validation of the client's experience and encouragement to integrate helpful skills at the moment. After reviewing the diary card and behavioral chain analysis, the therapist can introduce the first core skill of DBT: mindfulness. The therapist will provide psychoeducation of two core mindfulness skills, "What" skills and "How" skills, followed by an in-session mindfulness activity to practice. Mindfulness will be a crucial skill for Charlotte to develop, as it will allow her to tune into her emotional experiences when experiencing urges to self-harm. Without this awareness, it will be difficult for Charlotte to terminate NSSI behaviors. For homework, the therapist should encourage the client to continue completing her diary card and to practice one mindfulness activity each day until the next session.

Sessions four to five

The focus of this set of sessions will be distress tolerance. After reviewing homework, the therapist can introduce the role of distress tolerance in managing urges to engage in NSSI or other maladaptive behaviors. Distress tolerance skills will be reviewed, such as self-soothing with the five senses, improving the moment, pros and cons, and the STOP skill (stopping, taking a step back, observing, and processing mindfully). A body scan may be completed in session to combine the practice of mindfulness and distress tolerance, and to bring awareness to the role of physical sensations in emotional experiences. For homework, the therapist should encourage Charlotte to practice distress tolerance skills each day of the week in addition to completing her diary card.

Sessions six to seven

These sessions will introduce the goals of emotion regulation. After reviewing Charlotte's diary card and processing her experience with distress tolerance skills, the therapist will provide psychoeducation on the role of emotion regulation in reducing emotional suffering and viewing emotions as neither good or bad. Charlotte and the therapist will work together to identify common emotions and understand the functions of emotions. This could be done by reviewing her diary card from the past week and noticing themes in her emotions. Lastly, the therapist will introduce ways to change emotional responses by checking the facts, problem-solving, and opposite action. For homework, Charlotte should be encouraged to practice these skills daily and to continue writing in her diary card.

Sessions eight to nine

These sessions will focus on interpersonal effectiveness, which will be important for Charlotte to address her fears of disclosing her sexuality to her family. The therapist should validate the non-linear, cyclical nature of the coming-out process and be mindful not to pressure Charlotte to disclose her sexuality before she is ready (Ali & Barden, 2015). To balance this dialectic, it would be equally important for the therapist to explore interpersonal skills that will empower the client to embrace her identity by increasing her self-confidence with communication. Charlotte and the therapist will explore effective strategies for asking for what she needs, saying "no," and coping with interpersonal conflict. DBT skills such as DEAR MAN, GIVE, and FAST (see Linehan, 2014, for more information and worksheets on these DBT skills) can be reviewed and applied to Charlotte's struggles with her coming-out process. Role plays may also be helpful to apply and practice interpersonal skills in-session. For homework, the therapist should encourage Charlotte to practice interpersonal effectiveness throughout the week and to provide an example of her application during the last session.

Final sessions

Charlotte's last sessions will begin with a homework review followed by a discussion on what was meaningful to her about the past six weeks of therapy. The therapist should encourage Charlotte to highlight specific skills that she intends to practice from the four core DBT skills. At this time, it would also be important for the therapist to assess and determine if Charlotte needs further treatment. Depending on her clinical presentation, it may be appropriate to provide referrals for outpatient therapists who can continue working with her without the time limitation placed by the university counseling center. The therapist may also recommend on-campus organizations or resources for LGBTQ students, which will expand Charlotte's support system during her coming-out process.

Before approaching treatment from a DBT framework, it is important to determine the client's appropriateness given their presentation. For example, Emma may not be a good candidate for DBT due to her current state of readiness for change. She lacks insight into the severity of her behaviors and questioned why the hospital staff would not allow her to engage in NSSI. Emma's current commitment to treatment appears to be low, so she may also feel resistant toward completing homework assignments that are crucial for effective DBT work. However, Emma may benefit from motivational interviewing (MI), which promotes an egalitarian therapeutic relationship, develops discrepancies, rolls with resistance, and supports client self-efficacy (Miller & Rollnick, 2002). The transtheoretical model (TTM) would also allow the therapist to assess Emma's stage of change and build motivation (Prochaska & Norcross, 2001). Since she appears to be in the precontemplation stage, Emma may be most receptive to the counselor's empathy, validation, and willingness to "roll with resistance." In combination, MI and TTM may be helpful to counsel people who engage in NSSI by enhancing readiness to change (Kamen, 2009; Kress & Hoffman, 2008). Table 10.2 reviews how the four basic principles of MI can be applied to counseling with Emma.

Table 10.2 Motivational interviewing—The case of Emma

Basic MI principle	*Definition*	*Case application*
Expressing empathy	Building a strong therapeutic alliance with acceptance, warmth, openness, and understanding	The counselor can validate Emma's struggles by empathizing that school and chores may feel irritating and acknowledging that self-harm is the only thing that seems to feel helpful to manage uncomfortable emotions.
Developing discrepancy	Uncovering and addressing discrepancies between the client's behavior and their values/goals	Using Emma's personal goals for therapy, the counselor may notice discrepancies between what the client wants and her actual behaviors. For example, if Emma reports that she wants to feel more connected to others, the counselor may address the discrepancy between her goal of connection and the isolation that she experiences when engaging in NSSI.
Rolling with resistance	Reframing resistance to encourage movement toward change	Emma's behaviors are likely challenged by others often, including family members. The counselor can choose to roll with her "resistance" to change, and paradoxically facilitate her change process.
Supporting self-efficacy	Building client's hope that they can change their behavior	Despite Emma's current resistance to terminate NSSI, she may feel more open to learning ways to manage her anger to avoid getting into fights at school. Emotion regulation skills may then help her to better tolerate urges to self-injure. This enhances Emma's sense of control and helps her feel like she can meet her needs in a more adaptive manner.

Source: Miller, W.R., & Rollnick, S. (2002). *Motivational Interviewing: Preparing People for Change* (2nd ed.). New York, NY: Guilford. doi:10.1097/01445442-200305000-00013; Kress, V.E., & Hoffman, R.M. (2008). *Journal of Mental Health Counseling*, 30(4), 311–329. doi:10.17744/mehc.30.4.n2136170r5732u6h.

Cognitive behavioral therapy

Cognitive behavioral therapy (CBT) is an active, problem-focused treatment approach that focuses on reducing emotional distress while increasing adaptive behaviors in clients with various mental health problems (Wenzel, 2017). Although DBT incorporates elements of CBT, CBT has not been studied as considerably as DBT for NSSI (Gonzales & Bergstrom, 2013). However, several studies highlight the efficacy of CBT as a time-limited behavioral intervention for both adolescents and adults who engage in NSSI. In a study examining the efficacy of short-term CBT with adolescents and adults who had recently engaged in self-harm, participants who received CBT along with treatment as usual were found to have significantly greater reductions in self-harm, suicidal ideation, and symptoms of anxiety and depression, while experiencing improvements in self-esteem and problem-solving ability (Slee et al., 2008). Additionally, a study examining the efficacy of a new CBT treatment manual for self-harming adolescents showed significant reductions in self-harm, depressive symptoms, and trait anxiety (Fischer et al., 2013).

CBT theorizes that maladaptive or unhelpful cognitions are essential to understanding psychopathology (Beck, 1993). In the case of Jimmy, some maladaptive thoughts he may be experiencing are, "I am fine since I haven't made a suicide attempt in a long time," or "It's better to harm myself than to break something." From a CBT framework, these cognitions perpetuate the cycle of NSSI through minimization of his current behaviors and inability to consider alternative behaviors. It would be important to explore how these maladaptive cognitions relate to Jimmy's psychosocial crisis of generativity versus stagnation from Erikson's developmental theory. For example, Jimmy may be experiencing negative thoughts about his ability to contribute meaningfully to his home, community, and marriage, which is worth exploring in counseling. Despite his beliefs about mental health care, his agreement to meet for four sessions demonstrates some willingness to change. Therefore, CBT would be an appropriate approach to utilize on an outpatient basis, considering the potential brevity of treatment if Jimmy decides to terminate after four sessions.

The case of Jimmy

During the first session, the therapist should build rapport and provide positive reinforcement to Jimmy for his decision to come to therapy after his recent mental health issues. Since Jimmy reported that he does not believe in mental health care, it would be important for the therapist to provide thorough psychoeducation on the efficacy of CBT. After answering Jimmy's questions or concerns, the therapist will complete a safety assessment, discuss any recent NSSI behaviors, and create a safety plan. Lastly, the therapist will assess the extent of Jimmy's recent alcohol abuse and provide referrals for local Alcoholics Anonymous (AA) meetings, as well as Al-Anon or Families Anonymous meetings for his wife. For homework, the therapist can recommend that Jimmy attend an AA meeting before his next session to supplement his bi-weekly therapy and to encourage behavioral activation.

The second session will begin with a review of Jimmy's homework. If Jimmy did not attend the meeting, he and the therapist should problem-solve and consider what interfered with his attendance. This can be done by using a thought record, which allows Jimmy and the therapist to process the situation and consider the relationship among his thoughts, emotions, and behaviors. Thought records or impulse control logs (see Appendix L) are also helpful for clients to reflect on their thoughts, behaviors, and emotions leading up to

NSSI behaviors. The therapist will then guide Jimmy through some examples of cognitive restructuring to consider more helpful thoughts to include in his thought record. For example, Jimmy reported that he self-injured after an argument with his spouse a few weeks ago. Jimmy's cognition leading to the NSSI might have been, "It's better to harm myself than to break something." By encouraging Jimmy to restructure his thoughts, he can learn to replace his maladaptive cognitions with more helpful ones, such as "I'm angry right now, but harming myself will not help me or my wife resolve the issue." For homework, the therapist should encourage Jimmy to regularly complete thought records and to continue identifying alternative thoughts through cognitive restructuring.

During the third session, the therapist will begin with a review of the homework, including recent thought records and AA meetings. After processing his experiences, it will be important for the therapist to address relapse prevention strategies since Jimmy has an extensive history of NSSI and substance abuse and may not commit to more treatment after his fourth session. Using a CBT framework, Jimmy and the therapist will create a relapse prevention plan and identify warning signs. By identifying common, unhelpful behaviors, such as isolating or having a drink, Jimmy can develop awareness of his triggers and plan to reach out for help to prevent a relapse. Despite Jimmy's previous reluctance to include his wife in therapy, the therapist should gauge his willingness for her to join his last session. It will be important for Jimmy's wife to be aware of his warning signs to better support him in his recovery from self-injury and substance abuse. Together, Jimmy, his wife, and the therapist can process ways to sustain his therapeutic progress. Creating a tangible self-care plan to address ways Jimmy can support himself in each of his five life domains (professional, psychological, physical, personal, and spiritual; see Appendix O) will assist Jimmy in maintaining his therapeutic progress and allow him to remember all of the ways he can support self-care and coping while maintaining his sobriety and not self-injuring.

By the fourth session, Jimmy may either decide to terminate services or to continue outpatient counseling. Regardless of his decision, it is the responsibility of the counselor to assess Jimmy's current presentation, recent NSSI, and severity of his substance abuse to make appropriate clinical recommendations. For example, if Jimmy has continued to drink alcohol and self-injure, the therapist should provide referrals for local substance abuse treatment programs that offer residential, partial hospitalization, or intensive outpatient levels of care, and have the ability to treat him within a more structured environment. If Jimmy has been engaged and committed to treatment, the therapist may recommend continued outpatient counseling to provide ongoing support with his recovery.

Despite CBT's efficacy with treating self-injury, some clients may not respond well to the problem-focused nature of the approach. For example, the case of Dean presents significant grief and change. Dean is grieving the tragic loss of his partner of 20 years, who was his primary support with his lifelong struggles with NSSI. As his Parkinson's disease progresses, he engages in NSSI when feeling like he's "losing control" of his movements. In Erikson's developmental theory,

Dean would be in the ego integrity versus despair stage. As Dean reflects on his life, he may be feeling a lack of fulfillment without his partner. Therefore, an approach like compassion-focused therapy (CFT) may be a good fit for addressing Dean's self-injury and grief.

CFT is an acceptance-based, cognitive-behavioral approach rooted in evolutionary psychology, neuroscience, and mindfulness (Gilbert, 2009). Van Vliet and Kalnins (2011) discuss how CFT differs from CBT and can also be used to treat clients who self-injure. Since CBT involves identifying and directly challenging maladaptive cognitions, Dean may benefit from CFT's focus on mindfulness and nonjudgment to increase acceptance of his emotional experiences. Additionally, from a spiritual perspective, Dean is more likely to connect with CFT due to the importance of faith in his life. A goal of CFT is to help clients become more tolerant and self-compassionate, rather than emotionally avoidant (Van Vliet & Kalnins, 2011). This approach will not only honor Dean's grief process but will also allow him to accept his body's response to Parkinson's disease and resist urges to harm himself.

Conclusion

It is evident that there is a multitude of treatment approaches that can be clinically appropriate when working with individuals who self-injure. Despite their theoretical differences, the models presented in this chapter share a common goal: to help relieve the suffering of those who use self-harming behaviors to soothe emotional pain. It is important to reiterate that the limitation of studies due to the protection of a vulnerable population may create difficulty for clinicians working with clients who self-harm, as they are unsure which practice is most effective. When in moments of uncertainty, brief reflective interventions that get the client to open up to the possibilities of a life without NSSI can be powerful (see Table 10.3 for some examples).

Therapists must be attuned to several global factors when navigating the best treatment option for their clients. One may reflect on Maslow's hierarchy of needs as a starting point and determine whether the client's basic needs are being met at the time of treatment. If not, resource gathering is essential to prevent client relapse. Another key factor to consider is client safety. When examining safety, the therapist may assess the client's physical well-being and the likelihood of serious damage or death while injuring oneself. However, other issues related to safety are also vital components for successful outcomes. Abuse and/or neglect may impede the client's ability to incorporate adaptive strategies into their plan for emotional regulation following distress. Additionally, the presence of an active and healthy support system is important while the client processes earlier trauma and is implementing skills to replace self-harming behaviors. With the integration of the aforementioned concepts and the knowledge of several proposed theoretical orientations, the therapist can then make an informed decision on how to help the client build a new foundation for change and recovery from NSSI.

Table 10.3 Brief interventions

Reflection		
Working with NSSI is hard. Sometimes we may not be fully prepared, and that's okay. Just remember that there are brief interventions that you can use in the moments when you are unsure of what to do with your client. Then, make sure to do your research and fully assess and conceptualize your client so you can choose the best approach. Below are some examples of brief interventions you can use with the case studies.		
NSSI motivation	*Basic and brief intervention*	*Clinician response*
Jimmy: Self-punish	Talk about self-forgiveness and guilt. How do you forgive yourself or let go of the feelings of being imperfect?	"It sounds like you are blaming yourself for a lot of the problems that are in your marriage. What would it be like if you could forgive yourself or allow space to be imperfect? Can we brainstorm that together?"
Dean: Feel something and alleviate numbness	Identify alternate strategies to reduce the current emotional distress, even if they are not eliminating the self-injury; they will reduce the risk of harm (e.g., take a cold shower, eat a hot pepper, or put ice on the skin for 30 seconds). Or discuss ways to tolerate numbness temporarily.	"Can you tell me some methods which would enable you to feel something when you are feeling numb and empty, even if they have not worked before? Has anything ever helped in the past? Would you be willing to create a list of options with me?"
Sam: Communicate with others	Find ways to communicate your needs and what you might be missing. Practice ways that you can ask for help.	"I know your mom is not around much because she is working, but it is evident she loves you and wants to help. When you are upset, how can you ask her for what you need before you hurt yourself? Can we come up with a few realistic ways to do this together?"
Rhonda: Reduce emotional distress	Find alternate ways to reduce emotional distress and anxiety. Discuss ways to reduce anxiety (journaling, exercise, relaxation techniques).	"When you are overwhelmed with worry about what other people are thinking, your kids, or even your ex-husband, what are some things that you could try before you self-injure? Would you be willing to make a list and we can discuss which ones would be most helpful and why?"
Rick: Emotional expression and release	Allow himself permission to express emotions. Find alternate ways of emotional expression and dispel myths and beliefs related to self-view and the way others see him.	"If you were able to stop picking fights, self-injuring, and acting out, what would that be like for you? How would your life be different? Let's imagine you are watching yourself on video a few months from now when you are not self-injuring, what would we see in your attitude and personality that would indicate you are better?"

REFERENCES

Ali, S.S., & Barden, S. (2015). Considering the cycle of coming out: Sexual minority identity development. *The Professional Counselor*, 5(4), 501–515. doi:10.15241/sa.5.4.501

American Psychological Association (APA). (2002). *Criteria for Evaluating Treatment Guidelines*. Washington, DC: APA.

Anestis, M.D., Kleiman, E.M., Lavender, J.M., Tull, M.T., & Gratz, K.L. (2014). The pursuit of death versus escape from negative affect: An examination of the nature of the relationship between emotion dysregulation and both suicidal behavior and non-suicidal self-injury. *Comprehensive Psychiatry*, 55, 1820–1830. doi:10.1016/j.comppsych.2014.07.007

Beck, A.T. (1993). Cognitive therapy: Past, present, and future. *Journal of Consulting and Clinical Psychology*, 62, 164–198. doi:10.1037/0022-006x.61.2.194

DeCou, C.R., Comtois, K.A., & Landes, S.J. (2019). Dialectical behavior therapy is effective for the treatment of suicidal behavior: A meta-analysis. *Behavior Therapy*, 50, 60–72. doi:10.1016/j.beth.2018.03.009

Diamond, G., Russon, J., & Levy, S. (2016). Attachment-based family therapy: A review of the empirical support. *Family Process*, 55(3), 595–610. doi:10.1111/famp.12241

Fischer, G., Brunner, R., Parzer, P., Resch, F., & Kaess, M. (2013). Short-term psychotherapeutic treatment in adolescents engaging in non-suicidal self-injury: A randomized controlled trial. *Trials*, 14. 1–7. doi:10.1186/1745-6215-14-294

Ghafoor, S. (2008). Out of harm's way. *Nursing Standard*, 22(43), 61. doi:10.7748/ns.22.43.61.s47

Gilbert, P. (2009). *The Compassionate Mind*. London, England: Constable & Robinson.

Glenn, C.R., Franklin, J.C., & Nock, M.K. (2015). Evidence-based psychosocial treatments for self-injurious thoughts and behaviors in youth. *Journal of Clinical Child & Adolescent Psychology*, 44(1), 1–29.

Gonzales, A.H., & Bergstrom, L. (2013). Adolescent non-suicidal self-injury (NSSI) interventions. *Journal of Child and Adolescent Psychiatric Nursing*, 26(2), 124. doi:10.1111/jcap.12035

Gratz, K.L., Rosenthal, M.Z., Tull, M.T., Lejuez, C.W., & Gunderson, J.G. (2006). An experimental investigation of emotion dysregulation in borderline personality disorder. *Journal of Abnormal Psychology*, 115(4), 850. doi:10.1037/0021-843x.115.4.850

Greenwald, R. (2012). *EMDR: Within a Phase Model of Trauma-Informed Treatment*. London & New York: Routledge. doi:10.4324/9780203836958

Healey, A.C., & Craigen, L. (2010). An Adlerian-feminist model for self-injury treatment: A holistic approach. *Journal of Individual Psychology*, 66(4), 366–383.

Kamen, D.G. (2009). How can we stop our children from hurting themselves? Stages of change, motivational interviewing, and exposure therapy applications for non-suicidal self-injury in children and adolescents. *International Journal of Behavioral Consultation and Therapy*, 5(1), 106–123. doi:10.1037/h0100874

Kissil, K. (2011). Attachment-based family therapy for adolescent self-injury. *Journal of Family Psychotherapy*, 22(4), 313–327. doi:10.1080/08975353.2011.627801

Klonsky, E.D., & Glenn, C.R. (2008). Resisting urges to self-injure. *Behavioral and Cognitive Psychotherapy*, 36(2), 211–220. doi:10.1017/s1352465808004128

Kress, V.E., & Hoffman, R.M. (2008). Non-suicidal self-injury and motivational interviewing: Enhancing readiness for change. *Journal of Mental Health Counseling*, 30(4), 311–329. doi:10.17744/mehc.30.4.n2136170r5732u6h

Linehan, M.M. (1993). *Diagnosis and Treatment of Mental Disorders. Cognitive-Behavioral Treatment of Borderline Personality Disorder*. New York, NY: Guilford Press.

Linehan, M. (2014). *DBT? Skills training manual*. Guilford Publications.

MacPherson, H.A., Cheavens, J.S., & Fristad, M.A. (2013). Dialectical behavior therapy for adolescents: Theory, treatment adaptations, and empirical outcomes. *Clinical Child and Family Psychology Review*, 16(1), 59. doi:10.1007/s10567-012-0126-7

Mehlum, L., Tørmoen, A.J., Ramberg, M., Haga, E., Diep, L.M., Laberg, S., … & Grøholt, B. (2014). Dialectical behavior therapy for adolescents with repeated suicidal and self-harming behavior: A randomized trial. *Journal of the American Academy of Child and Adolescent Psychiatry*, 53(10), 1082–1091. doi:10.1016/j.jaac.2014.07.003

Miller, A.L., & Smith, H.L. (2008). Adolescent non-suicidal self-injurious behavior: The latest epidemic to assess and treat. *Applied and Preventive Psychology*, 12, 178–188. doi:10.1016/j.appsy.2008.05.003

Miller, W.R., & Rollnick, S. (2002). *Motivational Interviewing: Preparing People for Change* (2nd ed.). New York: Guilford. doi:10.1097/01445442-200305000-00013

Mosquera, D., & Ross, C. (2016). Application of EMDR therapy to self-harming behaviors. *Journal of EMDR Practice and Research*, 10(2), 119–128. doi:10.1891/1933-3196.10.2.119

Muehlenkamp, J.J. (2006). Empirically supported treatments and general therapy guidelines for non-suicidal self-injury. *Journal of Mental Health Counseling*, 28(2), 166–185. doi:10.17744/mehc.28.2.6w61cut2lxjdg3m7

Nock, M.K. (2010). Self-injury. *Annual Review of Clinical Psychology*, 6, 339–363. doi:10.1146/annurev.clinpsy.121208.131258

Nock, M.K., & Mendes, W.B. (2008). Physiological arousal, distress tolerance, and social problem-solving deficits among adolescent self-injurers. *Journal of Consulting and Clinical Psychology*, 76(1), 28–38. doi:10.1037/0022-006x.76.1.28

Pembroke, L. (2006). Limiting self harm. *Emergency Nurse*, 14(5), 8–10. doi:10.7748/en.14.5.8.s13

Prochaska, J.O., & Norcross, J.C. (2001). Stages of change. *Psychotherapy*, 38, 443–448. doi:10.1037/0033-3204.38.4.443

Rathus, J.H., & Miller, A.L. (2002). Dialectical behavior therapy adapted for suicidal adolescents. *Suicide and Life-Threatening Behavior*, 32(2), 146. doi:10.1521/suli.32.2.146.24399

Shapiro, F. (2018). *Eye Movement Desensitization and Reprocessing (EMDR) Therapy: Basic Principles, Protocols, and Procedures*. New York, NY: The Guilford Press.

Singhal, N., & Bhola, P. (2017). Ethical practices in community-based research in non-suicidal self-injury: A systematic review. *Asian Journal of Psychiatry*, 30, 127–134. doi:10.1016/j.ajp.2017.08.015

Slee, N., Garnefski, N., Van der Leeden, R., Arensman, E., & Spinhoven, P. (2008). Cognitive-behavioural intervention for self-harm: Randomised controlled trail. *British Journal of Psychiatry*, 192(3), 202–211. doi:10.1192/bjp.bp.107.037564

Stanley, B., Brodsky, B., Nelson, J.D., & Dulit, R. (2007). Brief dialectical behavior therapy (DBT-B) for suicidal behavior and non-suicidal self-injury. *Archives of Suicide Research: Official Journal of the International Academy for Suicide Research*, 11(4), 337–341. doi:10.1080/13811110701542069

Van Vliet, K.J., & Kalnins, G.R.C. (2011). A compassion-focused approach to nonsuicidal self-injury. *Journal of Mental Health Counseling*, 33(4), 295–311. doi:10.17744/mehc.33.4.j7540338q223t417

Wenzel, A. (2017). Basic strategies of cognitive behavioral therapy. *Psychiatric Clinics of North America*, 40, 597–609. doi:10.1016/j.psc.2017.07.001

11 Future research and directions

Kelly Emelianchik-Key and Amanda La Guardia

As you have read in preceding chapters, non-suicidal self-injury research and treatment have come a long way in the last 15 years. One of the greatest advancements in NSSI research came about with the inclusion of the category of non-suicidal self-injury in the Diagnostic and Statistical Manual-5, section three, which was the first step toward creating a uniform definition and criteria for clinicians and researchers. Previously, definitions of NSSI, deliberate self-harm and self-injurious behaviors were often used interchangeability in the research, and many terms were used to describe similar phenomena. Research is progressing our knowledge of NSSI behaviors, which allows for better understanding, treatment, intervention, and prevention efforts. There is still a lot we don't know about factors influencing the development and severity of NSSI and how those factors intersect with typical developmental concerns across the lifespan.

Conceptualization

Currently, NSSI is defined in the classification system of the World Health Organization (ICD-10) as a symptom of borderline personality disorder or as "intentional self-injury with a sharp object" (X78). The DSM-5 added NSSI as a probable independent diagnostic entity (NSSID) in section three, as a condition for further study. The definition also undoubtedly distinguishes NSSI from suicidality, and from the definition of "deliberate self-harm" (DSH), which includes all self-injurious acts, despite suicidal or non-suicidal intentionality. Adding NSSI to the DSM-5 was a leap forward in NSSI research, as it assisted clinicians and researchers by offering a consistent conceptualization of NSSI so that results can be compared and generalized more readily. However, there is still an ongoing debate regarding whether NSSI should be included in the DSM-5 as an independent disorder, which could significantly improve knowledge about the etiology, phenomenology, and treatment of NSSI and facilitate the use of diagnostic interviews, such as the CANDI (Clinician-Administered NSSI Disorder Index; Gratz et al., 2015). Currently, NSSI has been associated with several mental health issues, including anxiety disorders, depression, post-traumatic stress, alcohol dependence, eating disorders, and bipolar disorder in addition to BPD.

The way in which clinicians and researchers conceptualize NSSI needs further advancement to facilitate the consistent evaluation of NSSI across studies, creating a foundation for results to be more generalizable. Clinicians continue to misdiagnose and misconceptualize NSSI use by clients, with evaluative issues potentially more prevalent among male clients engaging in the behavior (Healey et al., 2010) due to gender-normative expressions of self-directed injury. Researchers, educators, and clinicians need to be aware of assumptions when conceptualizing NSSI behaviors with clients and work to gain a clear understanding of NSSI—identifying what is known about the behavior and what is still unknown. Practitioners may conceptualize this behavior in multiple ways depending on cultural factors present for clients. Heterogeneity in client samples and prevalence estimates lead to underestimation of the diversity of clients who self-injure, which in turn leads practitioners to look for a singular type of client when considering self-injury (typically White adolescent females). When conceptualizing NSSI for research studies, researchers need to explore the frequency, severity, and period between the self-injurious behaviors, so that results can be consistent, measurable, and clinically applicable with regard to assessment and treatment planning.

Along with functional conceptualization, it is important to gain a clear consensus regarding definitions of *current* and *lifetime* NSSI. Many researchers already utilize similar definitions, which do not entirely encapsulate the distinctions between these groups. For example, many studies do not distinguish between those who engage in NSSI later in life within the *current* group versus those who stop NSSI earlier in *lifetime* groups. These are important and clinically relevant factors to distinguish, as they potentially influence the understanding of both risk and protective factors as well as treatment outcomes and future directions for prevention and intervention.

Diversity

Ethnicity, gender, socioeconomic status, race, and sexual orientation are all sociodemographic variables that contribute to experiences that may influence NSSI risk and prevalence. There is some evidence that NSSI may be more common among Caucasian individuals in Westernized cultures, but this could be due to sample heterogeneity (Gratz, 2006) and population access for research. Many current studies do not report significant differences with regard to the use of NSSI when accounting for race and ethnicity even when comparison groups are available. As noted, some studies have shown that NSSI differs across racial and ethnic groups. Though findings are different across studies, more research exploring racial and ethnic diversity surrounding NSSI needs to be done to better understand cultural barriers for care, cultural perspectives regarding self-injury, and protective factors that might be present within diverse communities. Research is in development (as evident through conference presentations at the International Society for the Study of Self-Injury and the American Association for Suicidology), and recent studies exploring differences in NSSI prevalence among racial and ethnic groups also explore why these differences exist. Wester and Trepal (2015) suggest that cultural and ethnic belongingness could be a mitigating or protective factor for NSSI among various cultural groups, though this hypothesis did not hold true across groups in their study. Culturally specific concepts need focused research attention to understand why certain cultural groups are more prone to NSSI engagement and prolonged engagement (e.g., for instance, White individuals tend to report more NSSI than other groups in some studies). Biopsychosocial factors related to NSSI require analysis through a cultural lens to assist in determining risk and protective factors for differing groups of people, societies, and populations. Recognizing these factors will also assist in determining if the treatment approaches for clients who self-injure need adjustment based on culturally specific needs, values, and beliefs. For instance, not much is known regarding risk and protective factors for NSSI in non-Western societies or marginalized groups within non-Western nations, but we do know that the behavior occurs in countries across the world. Gholamrezaei et al. (2017) assessed NSSI in non-Western cultures to review similarities and differences regarding commonly recognized characteristics of NSSI in Western cultures. Importantly, their research indicated that other factors, like socioeconomic status and gender might mediate the role of race and ethnicity for NSSI. While prevalence rates, preferred methods, risk factors, and age of onset seemed similar between Western and non-Western societies; gender differences were less noticeable in non-Western cultures. They and other researchers call for more diversity in researched populations, societies, and subcultures to understand better the interactions of biopsychosocial and cultural factors as they influence NSSI behaviors across the lifespan.

Gender and sexual orientation

Gender and sexual orientation are two areas where a tremendous amount of research is still needed. Research demonstrates that clinicians may overlook or fail to identify NSSI for male clients, when odds of engaging in NSSI tend to be equal for males (Emelianchik-Key et al., 2016; Muehlenkamp & Gutierrez, 2007; Whitlock et al., 2011). We also know that NSSI may function to regulate emotional experience across genders, but we still need a deeper exploration of gender differences to understand how gender expression and norms influence function. The biggest challenge seems to be how to gain proportionate samples of men and women engaging in NSSI for comparative analysis. Adolescence is a developmental period in which gender differences become more pronounced and a time when NSSI onset typically begins. These differences between young males and females lead to unanswered questions regarding whether younger age groups are more likely to report NSSI engagement honestly, or whether males cope better and stop self-injuring as they get older.

Additionally, the role that stigma and gender norms play in NSSI function needs examination. More specifically, researchers must explore the topic of gender conformity and how it may influence the intra- and interpersonal reasoning for NSSI, methods, and the frequency, severity, and emotional experience associated with NSSI engagement. For example, males who adhere to strict gender roles may deliberately engage in physical fights, engage in more risk-taking knowing injury to self will result, and show more signs of aggression as a way of engaging in NSSI, adhering to expected gender roles (externalizing behaviors). Claes et al. (2007) found men reported engaging in NSSI as a sign of strength and offered rationales that included a desire "to show others how tough I am." Though statistically non-significant, results lead to more questions about how cultural gender roles and norms factor into the expression of self-injurious behaviors. If accurate, it indicates that boys and men may engage in NSSI for reasons that are potentially both emotionally regulatory and socially based, as opposed to purely internalized purposes. An exploration into gender differences in NSSI will assist in the development of new theories, help better explain differences in risk and protective factors, and possibly inform gender-specific prevention and intervention efforts to reduce NSSI.

Sexual orientation and sexual minority status and their relationship to NSSI warrant further study as well, as sexuality is intricately tied to heteronormative cultural expectations. Current literature has demonstrated sexual minority status may increase the risk for NSSI as compared to heterosexual populations (Cramer et al., 2016); however, beyond risk, there is little concrete information directly linking sexual orientation and self-injury. We do know that sexual minorities experience minority stress that is internalized and can cause maladaptive cognitions; however, it is not fully understood how to address this stress with regard to self-injury. Further development of evidence-based approaches and interventions to work with those who identify as a sexual minority would greatly benefit those LGBTQI populations who are at a much greater risk for suicide and suicidal ideation. Additional exploration of protective factors will assist in the ability to build resiliency while recognizing the clear societal oppression and very real danger experienced by this group throughout the world.

Socioeconomic status

Socioeconomic status has been linked to NSSI in several ways, but questions about SES and responses may vary depending on how the questions are phrased and who is answering. Adolescents may not have a clear understanding of parental SES or developmentally may have a different perception of finances when asked questions such as: "What was your family's financial status while growing up, poor or comfortable?" (Gollust et al., 2008). Answers to these questions need to be compared with school records, postal codes, or even cross-compared with parental responses. Those with homeless histories are found to be 4.1 times more likely to attempt suicide than those with no homeless histories (23.1% vs. 4.5%) (Tsai & Cao, 2019). Suicide has many overlapping risk factors and similarities with NSSI, so it would be expected that low SES and homeless populations would also be at higher risk for NSSI engagement, but there are no concrete or strong associations in the literature. Clearly defined information on socioeconomic status, the start of NSSI behaviors, active engagement status, and so on would assist researchers and clinicians to ensure proper assumptions and generalizations.

Assessment and risk factors

In order to properly examine psychosocial risk factors, researchers need to pay more attention to the assessment of current behavior so that concurrent risk can be explored. Additionally, when assessing for risk, more attention to specific aspects of NSSI behavior among those who self-injure within a brief period, compared with those with a history of NSSI, could assist in understanding these groups. Assessments and measures that incorporate specific items about NSSI in national surveys of youth (such as the Youth Risk Behavior Survey) could facilitate this effort and allow for greater samples to be accessed, as well as helping determine if people in certain geographic regions are more prone to self-injury. Assessments that specifically aim to examine protective factors associated with current versus lifetime NSSI would assist in gaining a better understanding of NSSI, as well as helping with intervention and prevention efforts.

Many studies that are available only use one or two measures of NSSI, and, depending on the assessment, some of them may not fully capture important information about the client. For example, some assessments only use a small number of items to examine NSSI, while others only intend to assess basic NSSI characteristics (specific NSSI behaviors, frequency, and severity). Lifetime and 12-month period prevalence measures should be provided to facilitate comparison of results across studies and to track prevalence over time. In order to improve reliability and promote honest responses, research should be conducted via anonymous self-administered questionnaires. Additionally, some assessments do not account for NSSI that happens in the greater context of other co-existing mental health disorders. Measures to assess NSSI and related disorders and interpersonal factors (such as bullying) are often self-reported and subject to recall biases. Multi-informant measures from family and teachers, as well as sociometric methods, such as peer nominations, may assist to address limitations of self-report instruments (Olweus, 2013). When examining the background, history, and methods of NSSI, checklists are often preferred over single "yes" or "no" items because checklists could trigger a memory of NSSI or an experience that the client originally could not recall. However, many institutional review boards (approving the ethics of research) and community-based settings oppose detailed checklists out of caution that they could encourage the behaviors, even though research demonstrates that asking about NSSI does not increase the risk of engagement or amplify distress (Deeley & Love, 2010; Muehlenkamp et al., 2010). Qualitative and more open methods of assessments are found to allow participants to contribute to research and to "tell their story" (Biddle et al., 2013).

Making sure that clinicians choose the appropriate assessment tools is vital, but NSSI assessment tools need to continue to flourish and expand with our changing knowledge and conceptualization of NSSI. Additionally, assessments need to evolve to identify the interpersonal processes that take place when clients transition from ideation to engagement in NSSI, as this period of change is critical to prevention efforts. There are many assessments that gauge the pervasiveness among those who already self-injure, but not among those who are having ideations of self-injuring. Those clients might still have time to stop themselves from actually engaging in the behavior, so spending time to do a complete assessment of self-injurious behaviors is imperative. This includes using multifaceted approaches with formal and informal assessment measures to fully gauge the problem, while also researching to ensure that the formal assessments are the most appropriate tools (Craigen et al., 2010). Additionally, some clinicians are utilizing home-based therapy services. If this is possible, it would be beneficial to conduct in-home assessments and interventions to find out more information on how the family environment may affect the problem. Due to the high risk of suicidal thoughts and behaviors for those with prolonged engagement in NSSI, additional importance must be placed on conventional assessment approaches and appraisal of interpersonal processes in order to identify at-risk clients before the NSSI becomes too pervasive.

Suicide

Individuals engaging in NSSI are at a higher risk for suicidal ideation and suicide attempts. The second leading cause of death in adolescents is suicide, and NSSI often co-occurs with suicide (CDC, 2017; Cha et al., 2018). But not all self-injurers attempt suicide (Joiner et al., 2012), which makes it imperative to understand and further research those factors that do lead to suicide attempts and completion. Several shared inherited factors greatly contribute to these associations. Research examining the mechanisms underlying genetic vulnerability and environmental factors, which shape expression and risk of progression from NSSI to completed suicide, needs to be refined. Preventing trauma may not be foreseeable, but engaging those in therapy directly after trauma could mitigate the risk of NSSI and suicide by reducing the liability of psychopathology. In addition, targeting pre-existing vulnerability factors could significantly reduce the risk of life-threatening behaviors among those who have experienced trauma.

Greater insight into suicide risk and prevention and intervention strategies could come from further exploration of psychiatric and socio-emotional processes that cause a potential risk for suicide attempts in youth and adults engaging in NSSI. Peer victimization and bullying have been prospectively linked to suicide attempts. Due to the pervasiveness of suicide in the adolescent population, it is critical to understand and further identify factors to differentiate between those who self-injure and think about suicide versus those who make attempts at suicide. Additionally, it is evident through the research that perpetrators and victims of bullying engage in NSSI. Thus, it would be beneficial to examine the differences and similarities in the contribution of bullying and Joiner's IPTS concepts of acquired capability with regard to both physical pain and psychache (unbearable psychological pain, linked to suicide). Longitudinal studies are needed to further examine and separate the concepts and connectedness of bully perpetration, peer victimization, and suicidal thoughts and behaviors. Peer victimization and bully perpetration are often reported together, which prevents the ability to explore differences among victims, bullies, and victim/bully combinations. Further analyzing how these concepts each influence the course of non-suicidal and suicidal thoughts and behaviors would be beneficial to NSSI and suicide literature. Additionally, enhanced understanding of other interpersonal stressors (such as attachment, depression, and trauma) that contribute to NSSI engagement and suicide attempts, rather than to ideation, could provide insight into preventing suicide.

Treatment and evidence-based practice

NSSI is a complex issue that is often linked to co-occurring disorders. NSSI is most often found within the adolescent population, but few treatments have been studied in this population. Most of the treatments that have an evidence base come from examining them in young adults. Self-injury is a problem that can start in early childhood and span the entire developmental spectrum. Specific treatments and interventions within various age groups need to be studied further. Dialectical behavioral therapy has shown some efficacy for adolescents and within group process modalities. Cognitive behavioral therapy has been studied as well, but no evidence base suggests that this approach is any more or less helpful in the treatment of NSSI than treatment as usual. Additional research regarding treatment and intervention is needed within all populations of self-injurers. Both experimental and nonexperimental studies of larger groups may prove beneficial in defining the comparative efficacy of the available treatments.

Schools

All school-based settings should develop NSSI protocols that meet the needs of their students. Schools need to provide more resources to: (a) identify those students who self-injure; (b) respond, assess, engage, and manage student needs; (c) provide education; and (d) make referrals as needed. It is imperative for schools to move in a direction that seeks to provide early intervention and prevention of NSSI behaviors. Having supportive principals, leadership, administration, school counselors, and mental health staff is indispensable for successful collaboration within schools to ensure appropriate care, given age of onset occurs in childhood. School administrators can often be hesitant to become involved in self-injury research due to concerns about reputational risk, NSSI protocols, social contagion, and the additional burden of workload and resources needed. School participation in self-injury research and prevention and intervention programs is a necessary part of ongoing collaboration between researchers and student communities to combat NSSI and get ahead of the problem (e.g., Groschwitz et al., 2016). Schools offer some of the most extensive intervention opportunities for those who engage in NSSI (Robinson et al., 2013). Conducting more research within school systems could further develop and improve theoretically and contextually informed intervention and prevention methods. Additionally, it can lead to refining what is known about the relationship between NSSI, the school, teacher connectedness, peer relationships, enjoyment of schoolwork, and perceived sense of control.

Teachers play a critical role in the school setting. They should be aware of practices that can enhance support among students engaging in NSSI. When possible, allowing for individual choices and initiatives gives students a sense of control. Additionally, providing numerous opportunities to experience success in achieving tasks and creating close and mutually respectful relationships with the students can help with NSSI behaviors (Ebersöhn et al., 2015). Schools can assist with NSSI risk by implementing socio-emotional skills and lessons. Research focusing on the importance of distinguishing between class and individual-level classroom climate will assist in determining if these factors play a role in NSSI engagement and contagion. School counselors and mental health professionals working within the schools should emphasize individual-level perceptions of classroom climate, as a negative perception of teacher support and peer relationships could augment the risk of resulting NSSI behaviors.

REFERENCES

Biddle, L., Cooper, J., Owen-Smith, A., Klineberg, E., Bennewith, O., Hawton, K., … Gunnell, D. (2013). Qualitative interviewing with vulnerable populations: Individuals' experiences of participating in suicide and self-harm based research. *Journal of Affective Disorders*, 145, 356–362. doi:10.1016/j.jad.2012.08.024

Craigen, L.M., Healey, A.C., Walley, C., Byrd, R.J., & Schuster, J. (2010). Assessment and self-injury: Implications for counselors. *Measurement and Evaluation in Counseling and Development*, 43(1). doi:10.1177/0748175610362237

Centers for Disease Control and Prevention. (2017). Suicide among youth. https://www.cdc.gov/healthcommunication/toolstemplates/entertainmented/tips/SuicideYouth.html (accessed December 23, 2018).

Cha, C.B., Wilson, K.M., Tezanos, K.M., DiVasto, K.A., & Tolchin, G.K. (2018). Cognition and self-injurious thoughts and behaviors: A systematic review of longitudinal studies. *Clinical Psychology Review*, 69. doi:10.1016/j.cpr.2018.07.002

Claes, L., Vandereycken, W., & Vertommen, H. (2007). Self-injury in female versus male psychiatric patients: A comparison of characteristics, psychopathology and aggression regulation. *Personality and Individual Differences*, 42(4), 611–621. doi:10.1016/j.paid.2006.07.021

Cramer, R.J., Johnson, J.C., Crosby, J.W., Henderson, C.E., La Guardia, A., & Stroud, C.H. (2016). Personality and coping styles: An integrated understanding of mental health among lesbian, gay, and bisexual individuals. *Personality and Individual Differences*, 96, 272–278. doi:10.1016/j.paid.2015.10.025

Deeley, S.T., & Love, A.W. (2010). Does asking adolescents about suicidal ideation induce negative mood state? *Violence and Victims*, 25, 677–688. doi:10.1891/0886–6708.25.5.677

Ebersöhn, L., Loots, T., Eloff, I., & Ferreira, R. (2015). In-service teacher training to provide psychosocial support and care in high-risk and high-need schools: School-based intervention partnerships. *Journal of Education for Teaching*, 41(3), 267–284. doi: 10.1080/02607476.2015.1044226

Emelianchik-Key, K., Byrd, R.J., & La Guardia, A.C. (2016). Adolescent non-suicidal self-injury: Demographic analysis of Youth Risk Behavior Survey (YRBS) trends. *The Professional Counselor*, 6(1), 61–75. doi:10.15241/kk.6.1.61

Gholamrezaei, M., De Stefano, J., & Heath, N.L. (2017). Nonsuicidal self-injury across cultures and ethnic and racial minorities: A review. *International Journal of Psychology*, 52(4), 316–326.

Gollust, S.E., Eisenberg D., & Golberstein E. (2008). Prevalence and correlates of self-injury among university students. *Journal of American College Health*, 56, 491–498. doi:10.3200/jach.56.5.491-498

Gratz, K.L. (2006). Risk factors for deliberate self-harm among female college students: The role and interaction of childhood maltreatment, emotional inexpressivity, and affect intensity/reactivity. *American Journal of Orthopsychiatry*, 76(2), 238–250. doi:10.1037/0002-9432.76.2.238

Gratz, K.L., Dixon-Gordon, K.L., Chapman, A.L., & Tull, M.T. (2015). Diagnosis and characterization of DSM-5 nonsuicidal self-injury disorder using the clinician-administered nonsuicidal self-injury disorder index. *Assessment*, 22(5), 527–539. doi:10.1177/1073191114565878

Groschwitz, R.C., Plener, P.L., Groen, G., Bonenberger, M., & Abler, B. (2016). Differential neural processing of social exclusion in adolescents with non-suicidal selfinjury: fMRI study. *Psychiatry Research: Neuroimaging*, 255, 43–48. doi:10.1016/j.pscychresns.2016.08.001

Healey, A., Trepal, H., & Emelianchik-Key, K. (2010). Nonsuicidal self-injury: Examining the relationship between diagnosis and gender. *Journal of Mental Health Counseling*, 32(4), 324–341. doi:10.17744/mehc.32.4.366740506r458202

Joiner, T.E., Ribeiro, J.D., & Silva, C. (2012). Nonsuicidal self-injury, suicidal behavior, and their co-occurrence as viewed through the lens of the interpersonal theory of suicide. *Current Directions in Psychological Science*, 21(5), 342–347. doi:10.1177/0963721412454873

Muehlenkamp, J.J., & Gutierrez, P.M. (2007). Risk for suicide attempts among adolescents who engage in non-suicidal self-injury. *Archives of Suicide Research*, 11(1), 69–82. doi:10.1080/13811110600992902

Muehlenkamp, J.J., Walsh, B.W., & McDade, M. (2010). Preventing non-suicidal self-injury in adolescents: The signs of self-injury program. *Journal of Youth and Adolescence*, 39(3), 306–314. doi:10.1007/s10964-009-9450-8

Olweus, D. (2013). School bullying: Development and some important challenges. *Annual Review of Clinical Psychology*, 9, 751–780. doi:10.1146/annurev-clinpsy-050 212-185516

Robinson, J., Cox, G., Malone, A., Williamson, M., Baldwin, G., Fletcher, K., & O'Brien, M. (2013). A systematic review of school-based interventions aimed at preventing, treating, and responding to suicide-related behavior in young people. *Crisis*, 34, 164–182. doi:10.1027/0227-5910/a000168

Tsai, J., & Cao, X. (2019). Association between suicide attempts and homelessness in a population-based sample of US veterans and non-veterans. *Journal of Epidemiology and Community Health*, 73, 1–7. doi:10.1136/jech-2018-211065

Wester, K.L., & Trepal, H.C. (2015). Nonsuicidal self-injury: Exploring the connection among race, ethnic identity, and ethnic belonging. *Journal of College Student Development*, 56(2), 127–139. doi:10.1353/csd.2015.0013

Whitlock, J., Muehlenkamp, J., Purington, A., Eckenrode, J., Barreira, P., Baral Abrams, G., ... & Knox, K. (2011). Nonsuicidal self-injury in a college population: General trends and sex differences. *Journal of American College Health*, 59(8), 691–698. doi: 10.1080/07448481.2010.529626

Part IV

Worksheets and resources

This section contains various resources that could be helpful to you or your clients in the process of treatment. Worksheets referenced throughout the chapters in this book are available for your use with clients. Feel free to utilize any worksheets and adapt as needed, as the activities within this book reflect adaptations of numerous counselors who have worked with clients engaging in NSSI. This is by no means an exhaustive representations of available activities meant to facilitate treatment of NSSI, but these are some of the most prominent and helpful resources available and are widely used in some form with those engaging in non-suicidal self-injury.

Appendix A: Resource list

Parents

Books

Brown, B. (2015). *Daring Greatly: How the Courage to Be Vulnerable Transforms the Way We Live, Love, Parent, and Lead*. Penguin.
McVey-Noble, M.E., Khemlani-Patel, S., & Neziroglu, F. (2006). *When Your Child is Cutting: A Parent's Guide to Helping Children Overcome Self-Injury*. New Harbinger Publications.
Siegel, D.J., & Bryson, T.P. (2016). *No-Drama Discipline: The Whole-Brain Way to Calm the Chaos and Nurture Your Child's Developing Mind*. Bantam.
Whitlock, J., & Lloyd-Richardson, E.E. (2019). *Healing Self-Injury: A Compassionate Guide for Parents and Other Loved Ones*. Oxford University Press.

Articles

Berger, E., Hasking, P., & Martin, G. (2013). "Listen to them": Adolescents' views on helping young people who self-injure. *Journal of Adolescence*, 36(5), 935–945.

Schools

Books

Juhnke, G.A., Granello, P.F., & Granello, D.H. (2010). *Suicide, Self-Injury, and Violence in the Schools: Assessment, Prevention, and Intervention Strategies*. John Wiley & Sons.
Martin, G., Hasking, P., Swannell, S., McAllister, M., & Kay, T. (2010). Seeking solutions to self-injury: A guide for young people. Centre for Suicide Prevention Studies, The University of Queensland, Brisbane. ISBN 978-0-9808207-2-0 Retrieved from https://www.mentalhealth.org.nz/assets/A-Z/Downloads/A-Guide-for-Young-People.pdf
Miller, D.N., & Brock, S.E. (2009). *Identifying, Assessing, and Treating Self-Injury at School*. Springer.

Articles

Berger, E., Hasking, P., & Reupert, A. (2014). *Knowledge and experiences of school staff towards student self-injury: Final report for schools and universities*. Monash University, Australia. Includes policy & flowchart. Available here: http://www.self-injury.org.au/

Bubrick, K., Goodman, J., & Whitlock, J. (2010). Non-suicidal self-injury in schools: Developing and implementing school protocol. Cornell Research Program on Self-Injurious Behavior in Adolescents and Young Adults. Available at http://www.selfinjury.bctr.cornell.edu/documents/schools.pdf

Hasking, P.A., Heath, N.L., Kaess, M., Lewis, S.P., Plener, P.L., Walsh, B.W., … & Wilson, M.S. (2016). Position paper for guiding response to non-suicidal self-injury in schools. *School Psychology International*, 37(6), 644–663.

Shapiro, S. (2008). Addressing self-injury in the school setting. *The Journal of School Nursing*, 24(3), 124–130.

Self help for clients

Books

Brown, B. (2012). *Men, Women and Worthiness: The Experience of Shame and the Power of Being Enough*. Sounds True.

Brown, B. (2007). *I Thought It Was Just Me: Women Reclaiming Power and Courage in a Culture of Shame*. Gotham.

Chapman, A.L., & Gratz, K.L. (2009). *Freedom from Self-Harm: Overcoming Self-Injury with Skills from DBT and Other Treatments*. New Harbinger Publications.

Clinicians

Books

Claes, L., & Muehlenkamp, J.J. (Eds.). (2014). *Non-Suicidal Self-Injury in Eating Disorders: Advancement in Etiology and Treatment*. Springer.

Eliseo-Arras, R.K. (2018). Addiction and self-injury. In: *New Directions in Treatment, Education, and Outreach for Mental Health and Addiction* (pp. 81–101). Springer.

Joiner Jr., T.E., Van Orden, K.A., Witte, T.K., & Rudd, M.D. (2009). *The Interpersonal Theory of Suicide: Guidance for Working with Suicidal Clients*. American Psychological Association.

Juzwin, K.R. (2015). *Daily Journaling for Self-Injury Recovery: A Therapist's Guide for Clients*. AuthorHouse.

Linehan, M.M. (2014). *DBT? Skills Training Handouts and Worksheets*. Guilford Publications.

McKay, M., Wood, J.C., & Brantley, J. (2010). *The Dialectical Behavior Therapy Skills Workbook: Practical DBT Exercises for Learning Mindfulness, Interpersonal Effectiveness, Emotion Regulation and Distress Tolerance*. ReadHowYouWant.com.

Purcell, M.C., & Murphy, J.R. (2014). *Mindfulness for Teen Anger: A Workbook to Overcome Anger and Aggression Using MBSR and DBT Skills*. New Harbinger Publications.

Smolinski, S.S. (2014). *Nonsuicidal Self-Injury and Motivational Interviewing in a College Counseling Setting*. Fuller Theological Seminary, School of Psychology.

Articles

Andreasson, K., Krogh, J., Wenneberg, C., Jessen, H.K., Krakauer, K., Gluud, C., … & Nordentoft, M. (2016). Effectiveness of dialectical behavior therapy versus collaborative assessment and management of suicidality treatment for reduction of self-harm in adults with borderline personality traits and disorder—A randomized observer-blinded clinical trial. *Depression and Anxiety*, 33(6), 520–530.

Kress, V., & Hoffman, R. (2008). Non-suicidal self-injury and motivational interviewing: Enhancing readiness for change. *Journal of Mental Health Counseling*, 30(4), 311–329.
Stanley, B., & Brown, G.K. (2012). Safety planning intervention: A brief intervention to mitigate suicide risk. *Cognitive and Behavioral Practice*, 19(2), 256–264.

Websites

Adolescent Self-Injury Foundation:
https://www.adolescentselfinjuryfoundation.com/resource

American Foundation for Suicide Prevention:
https://afsp.org/find-support/resources/

Autism and self-harm:
https://www.selfharm.co.uk/get-information/the-facts/autism-and-self-harm

Centers for Disease Control and Prevention:
https://www.cdc.gov/nchs/fastats/suicide.htm

Childmind Institute: Parenting Styles:
https://childmind.org/topics/concerns/parenting-styles/

Collaborative for Academic, Social and Emotional Learning:
http://www.casel.org

Cornell Research Program on Self-Injurious Behaviors:
www.selfinjury.bctr.cornell.edu

CRPSIR training page:
http://www.selfinjury.bctr.cornell.edu/training.html

International Society for the Study of Self-Harm:
https://itriples.org/resources/

Lifesigns:
http://www.lifesigns.org.uk/guidance-for-others/

National Institute of Mental Health (NIMH):
https://www.nimh.nih.gov/health/topics/suicide-prevention/index.shtml

Psychotherapy.net:
http://www.psychotherapy.net/data/uploads/5113d7e764eea.pdf
Narrative therapy with children from the series Child Therapy with the Experts.

Resources for addressing mental health issues in schools:
http://smhp.psych.ucla.edu/

S.A.F.E. Alternatives:
http://www.selfinjury.com/index.html

Substance Abuse and Mental Health Services Administration (SAMHSA):
https://www.samhsa.gov/find-help/suicide-prevention

TalkSpace:
https://www.talkspace.com/

TalkSpace is a digital therapy resource, allowing users to engage with a therapist anytime on their smartphone or through the web.

The Trevor Project–Trevor Support Center—Self-Injury:
https://www.thetrevorproject.org/trvr_support_center/selfinjury/#sm.001qxe0a61drpdibl 0vykdg96whas

The National Self-Harm Network:
(UK): http://www.selfharm.org.uk/default.aspa

The American Self-Harm Information Clearinghouse (ASHIC):
http://www.selfinjury.org/indexnet.html

Heart Math:
http://www.heartmath.org/about-us/overview.html

Self-Injury Outreach and Support:
http://sioutreach.org/

Appendix B: Elementary safety plan

My name is ________________________________ and I will spend time with my counselor and people I care about to feel calm when I am having a problem. This is the story of *the problem* and what I can do to keep it out of my life.

Today the problem is

____

(give *the problem a name;* name the problem whatever you want)

My problem asks me to ____ and
(what things does *the problem (name above)* ask you to do?)

this causes me to feel ____ and
(how do you feel when *the problem* is around?)

people may see me do ____ but
(what do you do when *the problem* shows up?)

sometimes I can ignore it; the last time this happened was when

____.

(when did *the problem* show up and you were able to do something different?)

I know *the problem* is around when I feel: ____

I know *the problem* is around when I think: _______________________________________

It helps me to ignore *the problem* when I do the following things:

1. ____
2. ____
3. ____

These are the people I can spend time with and/or talk to who will help me to ignore *the problem* when it shows up (school & home):

1. ____
2. ____
3. ____

These are the people I can spend time with and/or talk to when *the problem* shows up and I am not able to ignore it and feel like I need help (school & home):

1. ____
2. ____
3. ____

www.AmandaLaGuardia.com

When *the problem* shows up and I need help, I would like the people I ask to help me to do the following (e.g., just listen and let me talk, tell me a story, tell me good things about myself, etc.):

1. ______________________________

2. ______________________________

3. ______________________________

I like the following things about myself and my life:

1. ______________________________

2. ______________________________

3. ______________________________

Tomorrow I plan on doing the following things that I enjoy:

1. ______________________________

2. ______________________________

3. ______________________________

I understand that my counselor will give a copy of this story to the adults who live with me and that I will continue to talk about this story with my counselor. If I woke up tomorrow and *the problem* disappeared for the whole day, I would know it because:

____

____

____

____

(what would you be doing and feeling if *the problem* was gone forever?)

Date: ________________ Time: ________________

Counselor Name: ______________________________

www.AmandaLaGuardia.com

Appendix C: Narrative storyboard

Writing a story about your life can help you to see things in a different way a find new meaning. Write a story about a past experience that was challenging for you and be sure to note the personal strengths you can find within the story.

1. Time – When did the story take place?

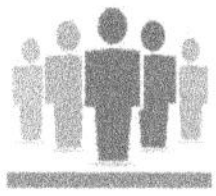

2. People – Who was involved in the story? What was happening for you and for each person?

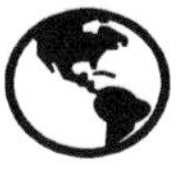

3. Location – Where were you? What setting were you in at the time?

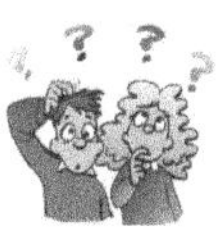

4. Problem – What was the problem going on from your perspective? If we asked the other people who were there, what do you think they might say?

5. Plan – What were your options in the situation? Looking back, were there other options? How challenging was it to develop a plan?

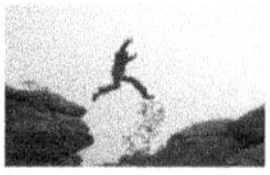

6. Attempt – What did you ultimately decide to do and why? How did you find the courage to move forward?

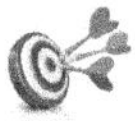

7. Outcomes – What happened in the situation? Make sure to note positive and negative outcomes.

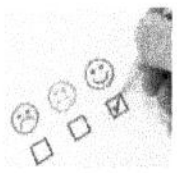

8. Evaluation – How did you do? How did everything end up? Looking back, what were some of the resources and strengths you used in this situation?

Appendix D: Cognitive mapping

Situation: Identify a specific situation where you repeat a patterned behavior

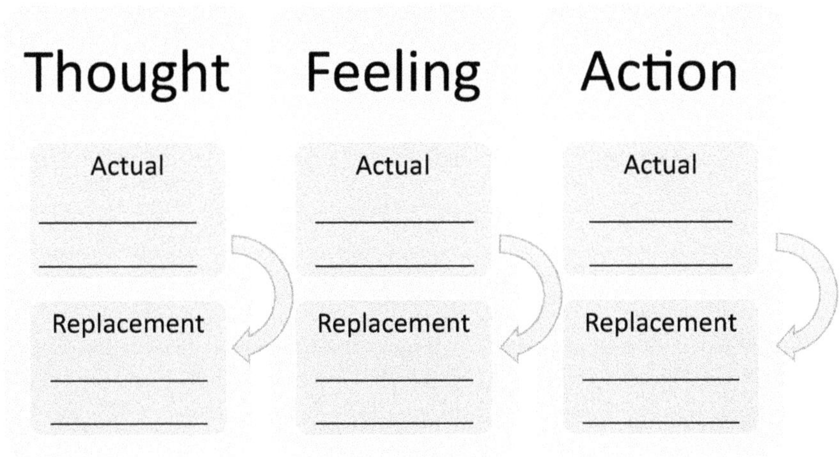

What will be the new result next time you run into a similar situation using your replacement actions?

Appendix E: Adapted DBT youth meditation

Set-up (Soothing Kit):

1. Bring some ice cubes for later.
2. Make some tea and drink a cup while you turn on calming music.
3. Turn on either orchestral music *or* forest sounds (rain, wind, etc.—**Relax Melodies app**).
4. Light a candle and lower the lights.
5. Wash your hands.
6. Get into comfortable clothes and sit or lie in a comfortable place.
7. Place a bottle of shampoo open beside you.

Close your eyes and bring your attention to your breath. Breathe in slowly through the nose, feeling the air move gently down the back of your throat, gradually filling your lungs. Feel the air expand your belly, bringing with it a cool peace. Slowly exhale, allowing your breath to move out from your belly and into the room around you, releasing a sense of calm into the space. Continue to breathe slowly, noticing the feeling of your breath inside your lungs, expanding your belly, and then releasing calm into the air around you. As you breathe, feel the air on your lips, your face, and then your skin. Allow it to embrace you.

Bring your focus to your body. Continue to breathe slowly in through your nose, and out through your mouth. Open and soften your body as much as feels safe to you and allow yourself to connect with your natural inner feelings of kindness and compassion for others.

Now, shift your attention to the wholeness of your being. Be present with yourself in this space. Now, imagine yourself lying in a comfortable place outside where you can see the sky. Feel the coziness of the ground beneath you. Begin to focus now on your emotions. Notice your feelings as clouds floating through your mind's sky, observing them, but not touching them. Watch as they float across your inner world. **(Pause for several seconds, slowly breathing and observing.)**

As you gaze upon your feelings, you begin to notice a breeze that brings with it whispers of thoughts in your mind. Refocus your attention on the breeze. Hear the thoughts. Allow them to pass you by without taking them in. Let them glide by you as you slowly inhale in through your nose and exhale out through your mouth. As the breeze of thoughts moves past you, you begin to notice how the wind feels upon your skin. Suddenly, the whispers are gone and all you can feel is the relaxing sensation of the breeze as it surrounds your body. Focus on that physical feeling. Listen to your breath slowly moving in through your nose and out through your mouth.

In this space, within your mind, you begin to speak quietly to yourself. Now you are in control of the whispers in the wind. You give it voice. You begin to breathe a new life into the sky with your words (include client-generated statements here):

"I am a strong, intelligent woman."
"I give my struggles meaning. My struggles give me strength. They feed my growth."
"My emotions give me purpose. I will use them to motivate me, they will not control me."
"While some people may not like my decisions, I know there are people who love me and will always love me."
"I will achieve my goals."
"I am a unique, wonderful person who deserves love and support."
"I love the person I am and the person I will become."

As you speak these words into the world, they begin to reshape the earth beneath you. The ground embraces you and fills you with a sense of peace and unconditional love. The sky above is filled with beautiful light, shining warmth upon your body, allowing you to feel a deep sense of belonging and acceptance in life. You know you are loved. You know you will overcome the obstacles in your way because you are strong and you have the support you need.

Now, keeping your eyes closed, slowly refocus your attention on your body. Notice the weight of your feet and legs. Notice the weight of your hands and arms as they rest. Notice the weight of your head. Scan your body from head to toe and notice any sensations you feel. Become aware of any tension that may exist in your body. Take that tension and imagine it melting away like ice on a warm day. Allow any tension to leave your body as you slowly breathe in through your nose and out through your mouth.

As you continue to breathe, begin to notice the environment around you. Bring yourself back into the room. Notice any sounds that you can hear. Try to notice even small sounds, like the breath entering and exiting your lungs, the sound of your own heart beating. Keep breathing and allow these sounds to become the focus of your attention. When you are finished noticing sounds, redirect your attention. This time, put your focus on your sense of smell. Notice any smells that are in the room. Become aware of the flow of air moving into your nostrils as your breathe through your nose. Allow the smells to join with the sounds around you to create a sense of welcome as you slowly open your eyes. Keep breathing slow, deep breaths. Take a minute to focus your visual attention on the room you are sitting in. Notice the objects in the room. Notice how light or dark the room is; notice the colors. Move your head to look around. Take everything in without thinking, without judgment. Allow any thoughts you may have to float away. Take five slow, long breaths and return your focus to the present. Return to your life with a new sense of focus, feeling relieved, safe, and confident in your ability to do what is needed to accomplish your goals.

Afterward (Use parts of soothing kit):

1. Smell the shampoo.
2. Chew on some ice.
3. Watch your pet play or attend to something moving (i.e., Newton's cradle) and count the movements until you feel ready to leave your room.

Appendix F: Bronfenbrenner worksheet

Directions: *For each circle, identify aspects of the person + environment fit that may influence symptom experience (thoughts, beliefs/values, behaviors, and feelings).*

It is recommended that this worksheet be integrated into your assessment process with the client and can be altered as an expressive arts activity with older children.

Describe the presenting concern:

- Individual—*Strengths and limitations, symptoms, role in relationships*
- Microsystem—*Family traditions and relationships, friendships, school/work environment*
- Chronosystem—*Generational trends and developmental abilities/needs/ challenges*
- Mesosystem—*Community networks and resources, microsystem interactions with community, social networks*
- Exosystem—*Socioeconomics (e.g., parents' work), extended family influence, neighborhood initiatives or trends (e.g., crime, resource availability, etc.)*
- Macrosystem—*Influences of cultural values, government policy, the economy, and other larger conditions, access to health care, and so on*

After completion of the worksheet, identify clinically relevant themes:

1.
2.
3.

What is your role in addressing these themes? What might need to be addressed through referral?

Place yourself within the client's system.

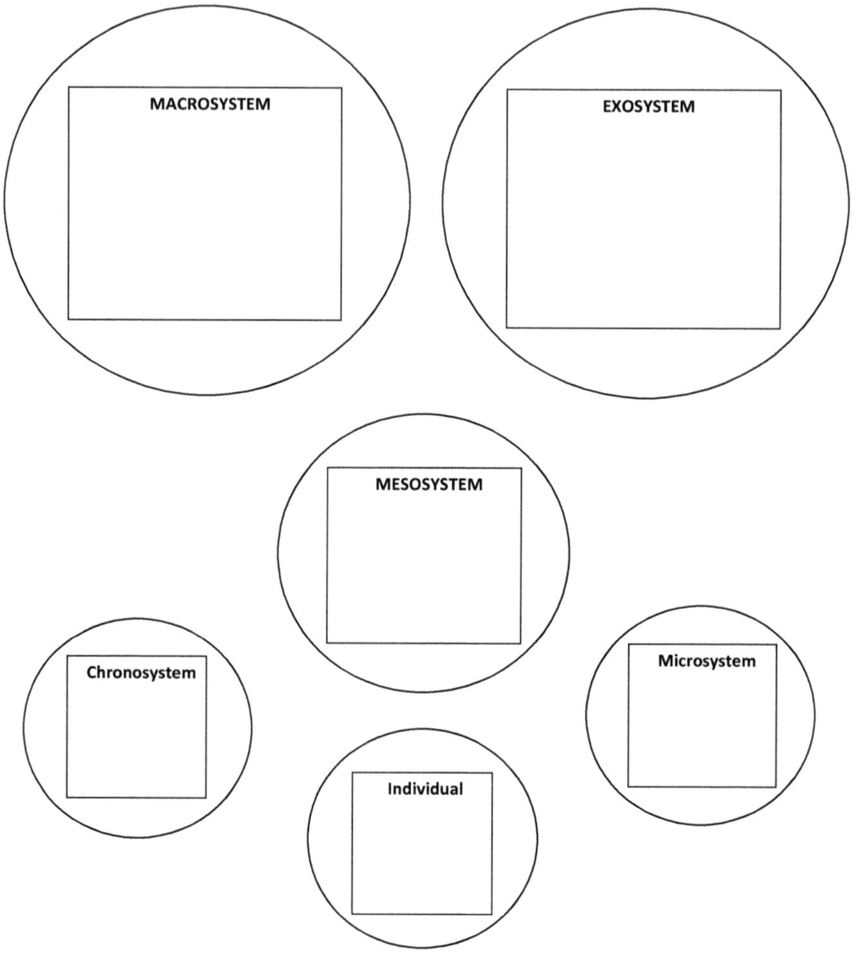
MACROSYSTEM
EXOSYSTEM
MESOSYSTEM
Chronosystem
Microsystem
Individual

Appendix G: Chain analysis of NSSI behavior

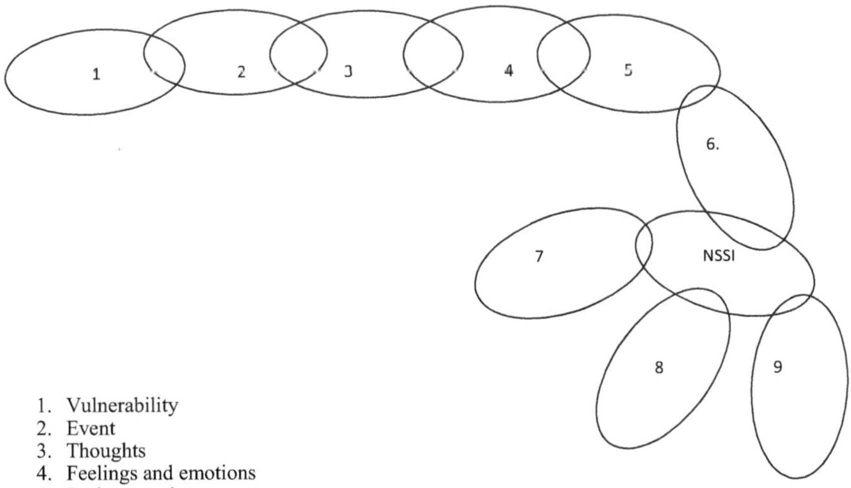

1. Vulnerability
2. Event
3. Thoughts
4. Feelings and emotions
5. Body sensations
6. Preparatory behaviors
7. Consequences
8. Consequences
9. Post NSSI/Behavior feelings and emotions
10. Ways to break the chain of events

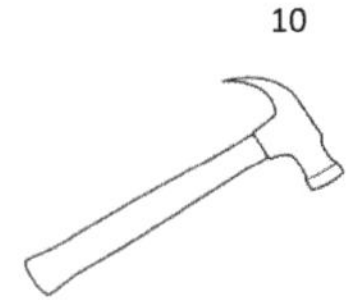

Appendix H: Checklist for working with youth

When working with youth in a community setting under the age of 18, permission for services is necessary from parent(s) or legal guardian(s). The consent process should include what information will be shared, what information will be kept confidential between the clinician and the child, and what the nature of that confidentiality will look like (as legal guardians/parents have rights to the medical records). This process should be done with the youth present. For more information about legal and ethical obligations, please see Chapter 10.

Initial Assessment

- ☐ Risk assessment: See "Severity Assessment," available through Cornell (http://www.selfinjury.bctr.cornell.edu/resources.html), and review the worksheet on risk assessment to screen for severity of injury, length of engagement, and suicidal ideation
- ☐ Family functioning
- ☐ Readiness for change

Family Involvement

- ☐ Level of caregiver awareness of self-injurious behaviors
- ☐ Caregiver link to use of self-injurious behaviors
- ☐ Caregiver interest in family counseling/involvement in treatment

Coordination of Care

Interprofessional collaboration

- ☐ Secure a release for the primary care physician and make contact
- ☐ Secure a release for school and make contact with school counselor/social worker

Safety planning

- ☐ Complete a safety plan (see safety planning worksheet)

Effective Areas of Treatment Focus

Based on the client's readiness, certain treatment interventions and protocols may be more effective than other treatments. Generally, each client should start by identifying the triggers that precede any self-injurious behavior and the process they engage in to feel better using self-injurious behaviors. One readiness-appropriate goal should be developed specific to the self-injurious behavior itself.

- ☐ Externalizing/naming of self-injury
- ☐ Assessing self-injury's involvement in the client's life (cycle of use)—*this is particularly important for clients who have been using self-injury to cope for three months or more*

Pre-contemplation or contemplation

At this stage, the client may not be ready to stop self-injuring due to a lack of other coping resources and an emotional reliance on the behavior. Thus, they may not perceive self-injury to be a problem. Thus, the focus should be on motivation and insight to support an investment in change.

- ☐ Motivational interviewing (e.g., "How do you see self-injury as a part of your life when you are your parent's age, if at all?")
- ☐ Recognizing how self-injury is helpful (e.g., "What does self-injury give you?")
- ☐ Recognizing when they have been about to cope without it (e.g., "Think of a time when you were not able to self-injure but you were struggling; what did you do to get through it?")

Contemplation and preparation

At this stage, clients recognize self-injury is a problem and would like to stop at some point, but are not sure what that will look like or if it is possible. Some of the same techniques listed in the previous stage may be helpful with some additions.

- ☐ Identify interests and strengths on which to build new coping strategies
- ☐ Identify support systems (see Wheel of Influence Worksheet)
- ☐ Self-soothing kit (one item to engage each of the five senses)
- ☐ Improve self-monitoring (explore situations in which client dampens positive affect)

Preparation and action

At this stage, clients are ready to try something new and will engage actively in a planning process and invest in trying new ways of coping. Behavioral techniques are effective at this stage, along with reflective interventions to assess effectiveness of new strategies.

- ☐ Relaxation exercise (See Mediation Worksheet—customize for client)
- ☐ Role play or sandtray (explore actual and ideal relational interactions)

Action and maintenance

At this stage, clients will be engaging in self-injurious behaviors far less or not at all and will be relying exclusively on new, healthy coping strategies. However, this stage is also tied to relapse. The counselor needs to communicate that relapse should be expected.

- ☐ Emotional regulation and acceptance groups or individual processing
- ☐ Distress tolerance
- ☐ Communication skills (see Communication Worksheet)
- ☐ Family counseling (parent-child relationship)

Relapse

This occurs when a client faces a stressor that served as a previous trigger to self-injury during the maintenance phase of change.

- ☐ Normalize backslides as an expected part of any change process
- ☐ Re-assess goals to ensure they are realistic
- ☐ Assess coping strategies

Appendix I: Building support circles

Dealing with challenges and conflict in the your family can be hard to cope with on your own. You will feel better if you can talk to other people about it. Think about the people you have in your life. Who can support you, and during what times might those people be the best ones to turn to? List family, friends, relatives, or anyone else who is close to you and is able to support you when things are upsetting at home.

Notice: You are the center. It is up to you to use these people who surrond you in your life and ask for support and help. Without you, the circles won't hold up.

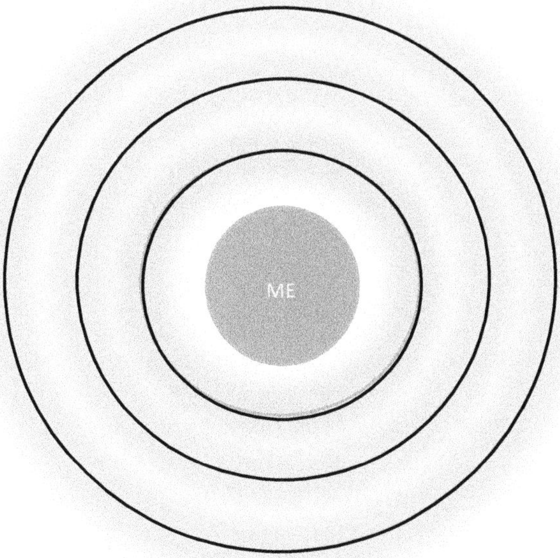

Appendix J: Taking your emotional temperature

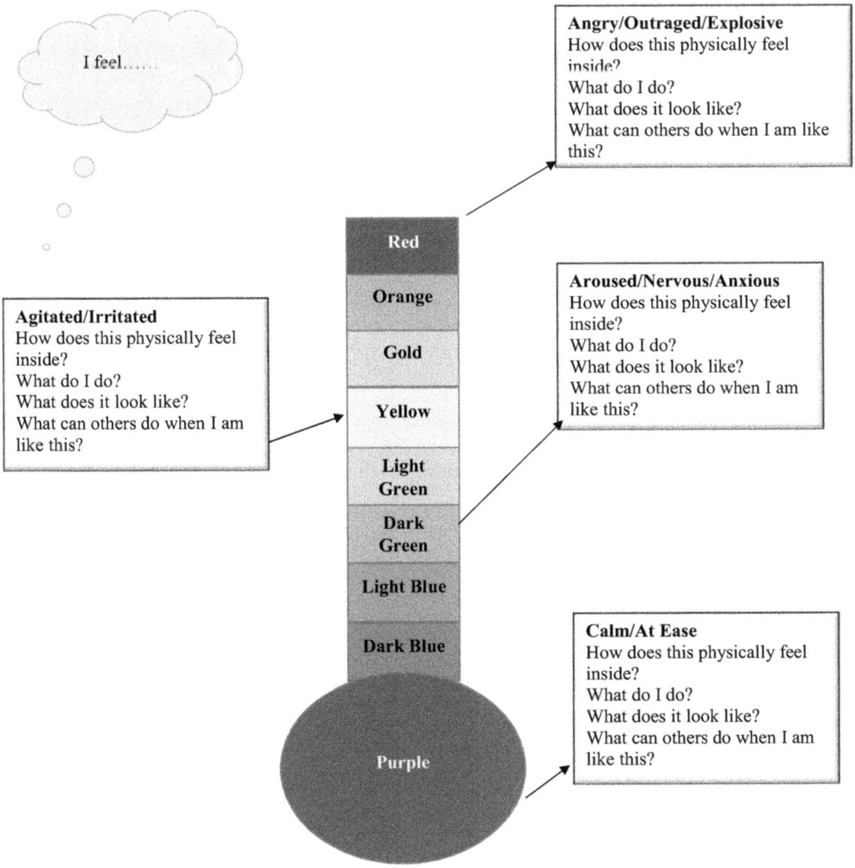

Appendix K: Voice of reason

Whenever you are having a negative thought about yourself or some aspect of your life, write it down. Then put it away. When you are ready (or in the moment), think about that thought and think about the *voice of reason*. What is actually a reasonable thought instead of your negative one? Remember, you are not expected to completely change your thought, but you can reshape it with the *voice of reason*.

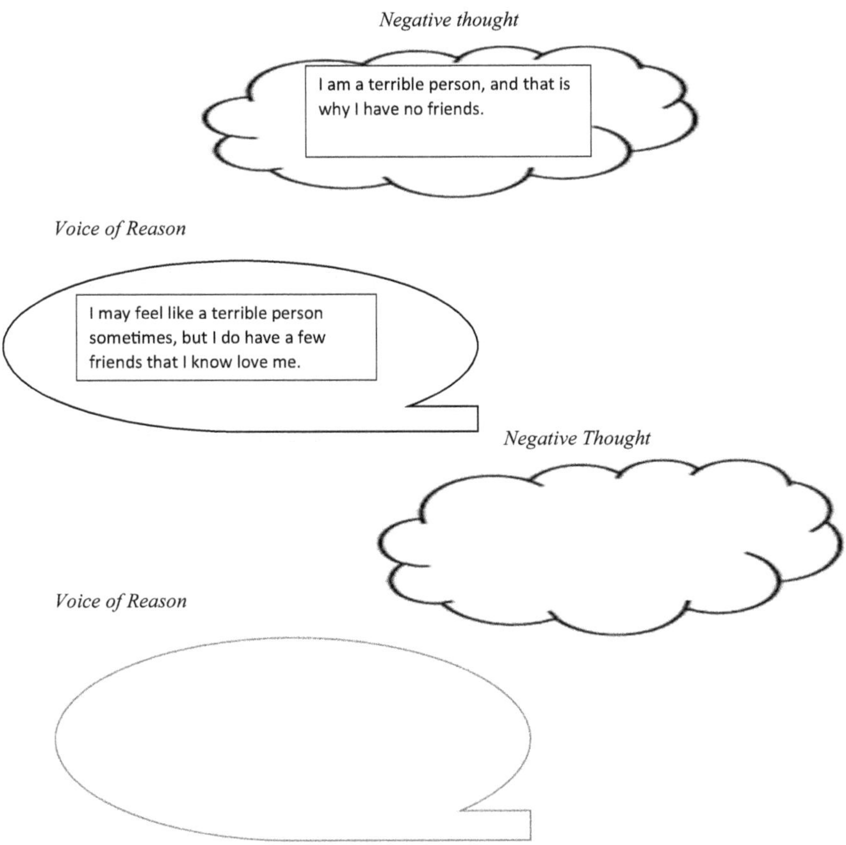

Appendix L: My impulse control log

Thoughts	*Time and Date*	*Location*	*Context and Situation*	*Feeling*	*What would SI accomplish?*	*What happened?*	*What would have been other outcomes?*
I am ugly.	11am 2/27/18	At the mall.	I was shopping for new clothes and looking at all the other attractive people in the store.	Ashamed, lonely, and embarrassed.	It would distract me from feeling like I am not good enough.	I was able to not SI until about 6pm by leaving the mall, but eventually self-injured when I got home and realized I never got a new outfit for school tomorrow because I was so worked up.	I could have put something together in my closet or called a friend to help me feel better. That friend likely would have let me borrow something to wear.

Appendix M: My life of purpose and meaning

Why are you alive?	
The thing that I am most proud of in my life.	
Who do you admire most in your life?	
What historical figure do you admire most and why?	
Looking back to a time before you retired, what do you feel like you forgot to prepare yourself for?	
If you could change the world in one way, what would it be and why? (Be specific.)	
What gets in your way of leading a fulfilling life and enjoying your later years?	
If people were to attend your funeral years from now, what would you *want* them to say about you? What can you do to make sure that this happens?	
When you were younger, what were three purposes you had in your life?	
Looking ahead, tell me three possible life purposes.	

Appendix N: Wheel of influence

Write your name in the middle circle. Write the names of those people closest to you in your life in the circles surrounding you. The farther the circle, the more distant the relationship. Write your name in the middle circle and then write two adjectives under your name that you think might serve to best describe you. After you fill each circle, write one adjective under each person's name describing how you think about said person. Write two or three adjectives next to each person's circle that reflect how you think that individual would describe you.

Example appearance below...

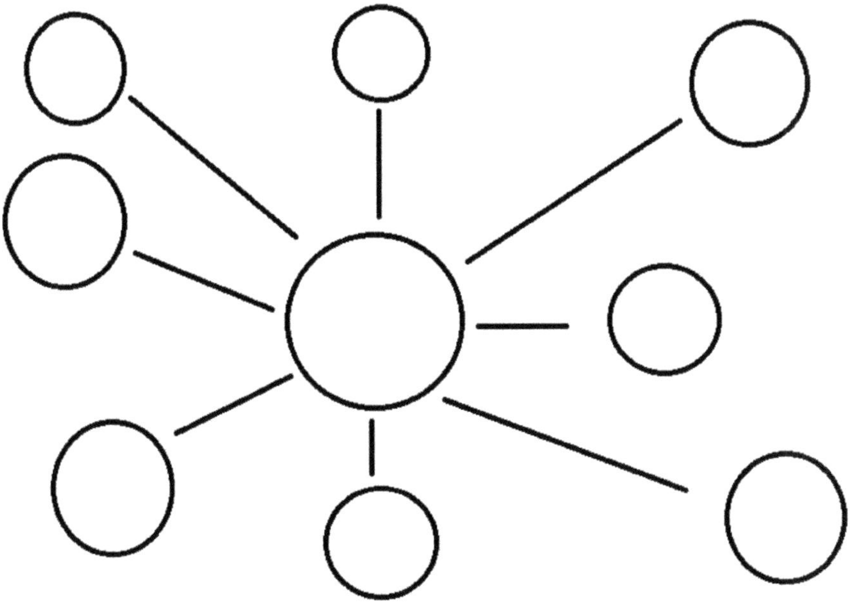

Appendix O: Self-care wheel

Self-care is critical to health and well-being. Fill in the self-care wheel with ways that you can support self-care in each of the following domains. It is critical to find balance in your self-care to support overall health.

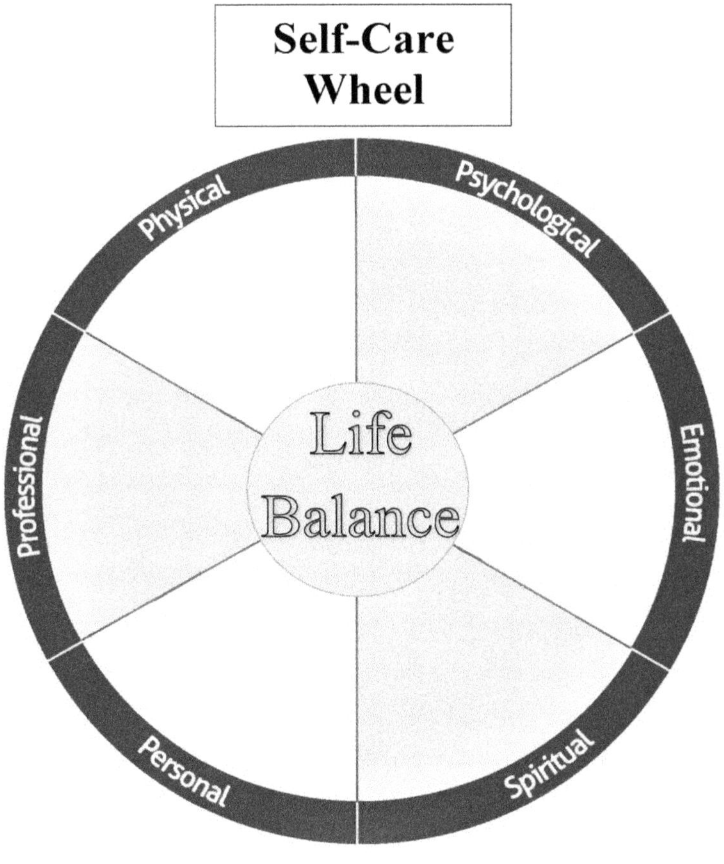

Appendix P: My house

When times are hard, it can be easy to forget the people and things that surround me. I am strong, and I have qualities that help me push through the hard times. I also have qualities that I want to gain. This is my house and it serves as my support, but as with all houses, it can be remodeled to always adapt to my needs.

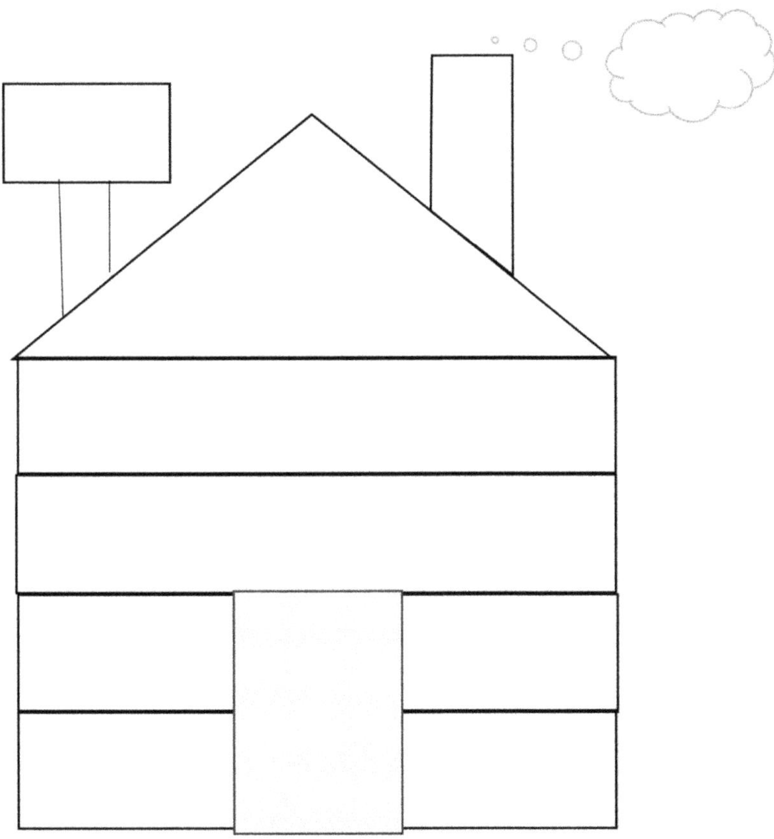

Parts of the House

Foundation: On the floor of the house, write the values that rule your life.

Walls: Along the walls, write anything or anyone who supports you.

Roof: On the roof, name the things or people that protect you and what do they protect you from.

Door: On the door, write the things that you keep hidden from others and you don't want people to see.

Chimney: Coming out of the chimney, write down ways that help you blow off steam.

Billboard: On the billboard, write the things that you are proud of and want others to see.

Levels of the House

Level 1: List behaviors that you are trying to gain control of or areas of your life you want to change.

Level 2: List or draw emotions you want to experience more often, more fully, or in a healthier way.

Level 3: List all the things you are happy about or want to feel happy about.

Level 4: List or draw what a "Life Worth Living" would look like for you.

Be as creative as you would like with your house. For example, is there anything else around your house, what materials are the parts of your house made from, and who maintains your house?

Index

Note: **Bold** page numbers denote Tables. *Italic* pages numbers denote Figures.

For Product Safety Concerns and Information please contact our EU representative GPSR@taylorandfrancis.com
Taylor & Francis Verlag GmbH, Kaufingerstraße 24, 80331 München, Germany

www.ingramcontent.com/pod-product-compliance
Ingram Content Group UK Ltd.
Pitfield, Milton Keynes, MK11 3LW, UK
UKHW022204190926
475702UK00003B/195
* 9 7 8 0 8 1 5 3 7 1 3 4 2 *